vised Edition

The Physician-Computer Connection

A Practical Guide to Physician Involvement in Health Care Information Systems

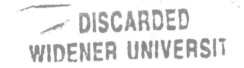

William F. Bria II, MD,
and Richard L. Rydell

AHA books are published by American H...
an American Hospital Association compan...

The views expressed in this publication are strictly those of the authors and do not necessarily represent official positions of the American Hospital Association.

Library of Congress Cataloging-in-Publication Data

Bria, William F.
    The physician–computer connection : a practical guide to physician involvement in health care information systems / William F. Bria II and Richard L. Rydell. — Rev. ed.
    p.   cm.
    Includes bibliographical references.
    ISBN 1-55648-166-7
    1. Hospitals—Administration—Data processing. 2. Information storage and retrieval systems—Hospitals. 3. Management information systems. I. Rydell, Richard L. II. Title
    [DNLM: 1. Hospital Information Systems. 2. Physician's Role. WX 26.5 B849p 1996]
    RA971.6.B75   1996
    362.1'0285—dc20
DNLM/DLC
for Library of Congress
                                          96-26417
                                          CIP

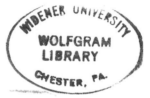

Catalog no. 093106

©1996 by American Hospital Publishing, Inc.,
an American Hospital Association company

Printed in the USA

AHA is a service mark of the American Hospital Association used under license by American Hospital Publishing, Inc.

Text set in English Times
2M—09/96—0437

Richard Hill, Senior Editor
Nancy Charpentier, Editor
Peggy DuMais, Assistant Production Manager
Marcia Bottoms, Director, Books Division

Dedicated in loving memory to our fathers,
Dr. William F. Bria, Sr., and Robert H. Rydell.

Contents

List of Figures

About the Authors

William F. Bria II, MD, is the medical director of clinical information systems and medical codirector of the critical care medical unit, asthma-airway program, and an assistant professor of medicine in the Department of Internal Medicine at the University of Michigan Medical Center (UMMC) in Ann Arbor. He has been a board-certified specialist in internal medicine and pulmonary diseases since 1982. Dr. Bria is responsible for the selection, design, and implementation of the Applied Clinical Informatics program at UMMC and has implemented a course for second-year medical students at the University of Michigan for the past four years. He has been a leader in educating physicians in the application of information technology to clinical practice for more than 15 years.

Dr. Bria is a fellow in the American College of Chest Physicians and a member of the American Thoracic Society. He is on the advisory board of the National Managed Healthcare Congress and *Healthcare Informatics* magazine. He is currently on the board of directors of the Medical Information Systems Physicians Association and is a past president of that organization.

Richard L. Rydell is president of the Keene Research Institute (KRI), a health care information management research, education, and consulting organization. Mr. Rydell cofounded KRI in 1992 to promote physician involvement with information technology and develop the Physician–Computer Connection Annual Symposia. He has been a leading health care chief information officer, serving as senior vice-president and chief information officer at Memorial Health Services in Long Beach, California, and vice-president and chief information officer at Baystate Health Systems, Springfield, Massachusetts.

Mr. Rydell is a fellow in the American College of Healthcare Executives, and is a fellow, past board member, and past national president of the Healthcare Information and Management Systems Society. He has served as an executive board member of the Center for Healthcare Information Management, a founder, trustee, and vice chairman of the College of Healthcare Information Management Executives (CHIME), and chairman of the CHIME Institute. Mr. Rydell is a charter member of the Health Information Systems Executive Association and a past international board member of the Society for Information Management.

Preface

It is rare to have the opportunity to fundamentally change the direction of one's life. To begin to see one's dreams fulfilled is rarer still. This book is the result of an opportunity that presented itself to the authors seven years ago. That opportunity has led to some of the most exciting and productive years of our lives.

In 1982, Dr. William Bria began working at Baystate Medical Center (BMC) in Springfield, Massachusetts, as a staff pulmonary physician. That same year Richard Rydell was working at Stanford University Hospital in Palo Alto, California. Their collaboration began three years later.

In 1985, BMC was an 850-bed tertiary care hospital with a proud history and a bright future. It was a level 1 trauma center and had an active medical staff of 450 physicians. There were 160 physicians in training in all of the major medical specialties, and the hospital was fiscally sound and emerging as the premier medical center in western Massachusetts.

Dr. Bria had been involved in several computer-interest groups for physicians since joining the staff at BMC. The purpose of these groups was to allow physicians to express their views on how computers could assist them in their day-to-day duties. However, each group seemed to fail when it came to the point of action. Time and time again, there was an initial flurry of interest from a group of physicians, and some interest from the hospital administration, yet nothing seemed to grow from these encounters.

Finally, in 1985, the BMC rumor mill revealed that the hospital was about to embark on the selection and implementation of a new "clinical" information system. After eight years of working with a "build-it-yourself" computer system, it was rumored that the hospital was considering changing direction, even hiring a new director of information systems.

To Dr. Bria, it seemed the time to act. It was time to find out whether the medical staff was really interested in using computer systems and whether the administration was willing to let them be involved. The ruling body of the medical staff was the executive council, so Dr. Bria decided to present the case to this physician council. The presentation allowed that there was an opportunity for the physicians to be more involved this time around with the selection of a system that really did something for them and their patients' care. The response from the physician council was a unanimous "Yes! We want to be involved." Furthermore, the president of the medical staff appointed Dr. Bria as the representative to the administration to deliver this message and report progress back to the council on a regular basis. A letter from the medical staff to the administration was drafted by Dr. Bria and mailed to the chief executive officer and to the information systems administration of the hospital. Dr. Bria was hopeful that this "note in a bottle" would reach the right people, but he was still unsure whether a real opportunity for change was at hand.

While these events were taking place, Rydell was thinking about rekindling his vision of physician usage of computers. Years before, Rydell had worked at El Camino Hospital in Mountain View, California, where he managed the implementation of a direct-physician-usable patient care information system. He then left information systems to become a hospital administrator, fully expecting the El Camino model of physician usage of computers to be propagated throughout the health care field. Ten years later he was very disappointed to find that the vision had not been propagated far at all. It was a challenge that he wanted to tackle again, for he felt that it was the right thing to do.

Two weeks later Rydell came to Dr. Bria's office to introduce himself as the new chief information officer at BMC, and to discuss the letter Dr. Bria had sent. Rydell indicated that the only way to select, design, and implement a clinical information system directed at improving the quality of patient care was to involve physicians in the project. Dr. Bria responded that he certainly was interested in such a project but that time was a problem — he was already busy as a clinician and as medical director of pulmonary rehabilitation, and he was involved in several education and research projects. At this point, Rydell suggested that he would be willing to pay for as much time as Dr. Bria could give him, so long as Dr. Bria continued primarily as a clinician. "I was shocked," Dr. Bria recalls. "You mean this is going to be an honest-to-God job?" "Absolutely," replied Rydell. A quarter-time position sounded "safe" and was agreeable to both parties at that point.

What followed was a period of testing and evaluation, although no formal process was visible to the casual observer. During this time, Dr. Bria remained somewhat suspicious that this information systems administrator might just be trying to placate the medical staff and not really provide the necessary authority to his position to make a difference. On the other hand, Rydell was concerned whether this physician was a valid representative of the medical staff, not simply a "computernik" interested in playing with machines and unable to see and accept the vision of physicians actually using information instruments to improve patient care. But the more each person saw of the other, the more each became convinced that the right choice had been made.

Dr. Bria spent the next year meeting with the medical staff and residents at BMC, visiting hospitals that had installed effective patient care information systems, and attending symposia involving applied medical information technology. He also gave lectures on how physicians wanted to be empowered to participate in hospital information systems projects, and how such participation could be advantageous for physicians, administrators, and patients alike. It rapidly became obvious to Dr. Bria that this was another full-time job, and he increased his time commitment to 50 percent.

In February 1991, BMC activated its patient care information system. The system is currently being used by more than 280 staff, attending, and resident physicians for order entry and results reporting on a daily basis.

Dr. Bria subsequently accepted positions as medical director of clinical information systems and as medical director of the critical care medical unit at the University of Michigan in Ann Arbor. Today Rydell is president of the Keene Research Institute, in Keene, New Hampshire. Their collaboration continues in national meetings, in the Physician–Computer Connection annual symposia, and in the book you are about to read.

Acknowledgments

The authors wish to thank Edwin Hawkins, Charles Cowen, Richard Linneweh, and Neilson Buchanan, hospital executives; Ralph Watson, MD, Margo Cook, RN, and Marilyn Davis, RN, clinicians; John Gall, John Fleming, and Chuck Olson, management engineers; and Mel Hodge and Bill Childs, product developers, for their vision, leadership, and enthusiastic spirit in pioneering the clinical use of hospital information systems.

We also thank Doug McConnell, MD, Harris Stutman, MD, Jack Ehrhart, MD, Malcolm Gleser, MD, John Glaser, PhD, John Teich, MD, and the many other medical informatics specialists who participate in the Physician–Computer Connection symposia. Special thanks to Kathy Larson, Jamie Barrett, and the staff of the Coeur D'Alene Resort, Coeur D'Alene, Idaho, for hosting the annual summer forum.

We especially wish to thank Michael Daly, president of Baystate Health Systems, Springfield, Massachusetts; Anthony Mott, executive vice-president; and Dr. Martin Broder, chairman of the Department of Medicine at Baystate Medical Center, for encouraging us to pursue new opportunities and for acting as coaches, counselors, and most of all, friends. We also wish to thank Dr. Fernando Martinez and Dr. Charles Watts for supporting a busy pulmonary service and for much personal encouragement; Paul Vegoda for being a friend and believer in "the connection"; and Rick Hill, senior editor at American Hospital Publishing, for his valuable assistance in writing this book. We would like to acknowledge our wives, Lee Bria and Sandee Rydell; our wonderful children and their families, Bill and James Bria; Wendy, John, Richie, and Emma Kipp; Vicki, Jim, and Anna Gottardi; Libby and Tom Dietz; and Rod and Jill Rydell; and our mothers, Dorothy Bria and Helen Rydell, for their love, support, and inspiration.

Introduction: Why Physicians Should Be Involved in Information Systems

Before beginning to consider why physicians should become involved with the design and use of information systems, take the following quick test. Pick up the latest copy of your favorite health care information system (HCIS) magazine. Flip through the pages to either an ad for an HCIS or an article about one. Look for the following claims, either directly stated or clearly implied:

1. Improves the quality of patient care
2. Improves the efficiency of care delivery and decreases costs
3. Promotes physician involvement because it is easy to use

Did you find all three claims? Now call five chief executive officers, chief financial officers, chief information officers, vice-presidents of information systems, or directors of data processing at five different health care organizations, and ask them whether their medical staff uses their HCIS and is happy with it. Not too many happy people out there, are there?

For many years, physician involvement in HCISs has been the Holy Grail of health care information managers. Most of these managers have realized that clinical benefits can most effectively be realized by putting the information tool directly into the hands of physicians, the leaders of the patient care team. Unfortunately, most health care information managers have been about as successful as Monty Python in reaching that Grail. This book is intended for health care professionals who are interested in defining, planning for, and achieving physician involvement in, and acceptance and use of, their HCIS to achieve tangible benefits.

Forces Influencing the Level of Physician Involvement

In any given health care organization there is a balance of forces influencing the level of physician involvement in its information system. Consider the following negative and positive factors contributing to that balance:

1

- *Fear.* This is principally the fear of change and is the same inertial force inhibiting all change in health care and clinical practice. It encompasses the fear of losing control and of losing confidence in one's own leadership position as a physician. Unfortunately, terms such as *computer literacy* have encouraged this kind of fear; grown, educated, and otherwise quite literate adults can feel inadequate and childlike in the face of the challenge of learning about computer systems.
- *Indifference.* Physicians are not professional computer users, nor do most of them wish to be. Their general lack of enthusiasm for technological wonders is often misinterpreted by data processing personnel as resistance. However, in reality, it simply underscores that physicians find computer technology interesting only to the extent that they can be persuaded that it improves clinical practice effectiveness and efficiency.
- *Inertia, or taking the easy way out.* The power of inertia is probably the greatest negative factor inhibiting physician commitment to a patient care information system. As the saying goes, "The more things change, the more they stay the same." The physician champion, introduced later in this book, is primarily a change agent who must overcome this force by means of education and peer pressure.
- *Degree of direct access to the system.* All involved in the design and implementation of an HCIS must share the expectation that to achieve its full clinical, patient care benefits, physicians must have direct access to, and make effective use of, the system. This factor is a powerful positive force for physician commitment because it reveals that the improvement in practice effectiveness and efficiency will be directly proportional to the number of active physicians using the system in day-to-day practice. For example, the more physicians actively using the information system for order entry, the greater the value of the electronic record to physicians reviewing it for details of care and clinical decision making.
- *Degree of cooperation between the hospital and the medical staff.* When a medical staff truly believes it is entering a partnership with the health care enterprise for the selection and development of a patient-centered information system, constructive energy is directed toward collaborating to meet that goal, rather than spending time and effort on resisting change and fearing loss of control.

The level of physician involvement generally falls into one of three major categories: oversight, casual commitment, or full commitment. The final balance of forces dictating which of these three categories of physician involvement is present in any given institution directly correlates with the preexisting relationship between health care administrators and medical staff.

Oversight refers to physician involvement at the most superficial level, that is, approving the enterprise's decision to obtain an HCIS but declining to become involved in its selection, design, implementation, or use. Although oversight fulfills the requirement for a physician representative on a planning committee, obviously this category of involvement is little better than no physician involvement at all. Then why include it here? Unfortunately, this level of involvement is far more common than the other two.

Casual commitment may be defined as passive physician use of systems that are normally implemented by other members of the organization's staff (for example, the nursing department, the data processing staff, and so forth). This category of physician involvement includes those situations in which the medical staff was informed after an HCIS was installed that "the computer is there to use if you want to." Most medical staff members walk away from such "opportunities."

Casual commitment can often take the form of *deferred involvement.* That is, physicians are only too happy to have the nursing department, students, and others use the information system in their stead. Deferred involvement is a common reaction among some physicians and completely obviates achieving the full clinical benefits of an HCIS because the tool is not in the hands of the primary users. The full consequences of deferred involvement become clear when answers to the following questions are pondered:

Question: What generates costs, uses resources, and determines patient care?
Answer: Orders.

Question: Who generates these orders?
Answer: Physicians.

Question: Who are the primary intended users of most HCIS installations?
Answer: Secretaries and financial departments.

Question: Who loses when it is recognized that the intended benefits of the HCIS have never been realized?
Answer: Everybody.

Casual commitment, therefore, is not acceptable in institutions seeking to behave responsibly with regard to their costs and the use of their resources.

Full commitment refers to the involvement of clinically important physicians in the process of selecting, designing, and implementing a hospital's HCIS as well as involving all physicians in its use. Full functional use of the HCIS would involve all clinical activities, including orders and results retrieval. Without question, achieving this category of physician involvement requires greater initial resource investment, risk, and planning. However, the benefits are clinical, financial, and operational. The balance of this book shows how to attain full commitment.

Why Physicians Need to Make Use of Information Systems

It is a reality of the practice of medicine in U.S. hospitals and clinics that physicians are at the top of the clinical decision-making hierarchy. In a very real sense, physicians are the managers of an ever-growing health care team, particularly when dealing with hospitalized patients. The communication and integration of information is as important to physician health care managers as it is to business managers (and, some might argue, a matter of life and death!), but unfortunately, the benefits of information systems that business managers have claimed have not been realized by physician managers. Most physicians are still left with the telephone and written charts as their principal resources.

No one questions the importance of bringing the latest medications and techniques to physicians for application to patient care. In particular, with the high costs of health care and health care reform a frequent item in the news, physicians are called on to play a significant role in controlling spending. Thus they need cost-of-care information at the time that clinical and cost decisions are being made.

The El Camino Story

Only a handful of institutions have been successful in providing cost-of-care information as part of their efforts to achieve the full commitment of the medical staff to using information systems. One such institution is El Camino Hospital, a 464-bed, not-for-profit, acute care, full-service hospital located in Mountain View, California.

Background

In the early 1970s, El Camino Hospital was the site of extraordinary achievements in information systems. Also located in the same community on the San Francisco peninsula was Lockheed Missiles and Space Corporation, which had developed a product that would later be acquired by the Technicon Corporation and renamed the Technicon Medical Information System (TMIS).

The publicly elected board and the chief executive officer (CEO) of El Camino Hospital had arranged with Lockheed to be the development and test site for the first fully integrated, comprehensive HCIS. Although it was clear that improvements in the delivery of patient care were a prime objective of the Lockheed–El Camino endeavor, it was also understood that the cost of delivering better patient care could be substantially reduced by eliminating errors and improving the accuracy, timeliness, and accessibility of patient-related information.

The goal of cost-effective health care was tangibly demonstrated by the agreement between the two parties: El Camino would pay Lockheed a monthly fee for use of the HCIS only if the hospital was indeed able to achieve cost reductions. In essence, the hospital agreed to pay only what it could save, to a maximum cap, and would and did recoup additional savings. This approach meant minimal financial risk to the hospital and contributed to the success of the project, as time after time, during the stress and strain of system development and implementation, the hospital board, administration, medical staff, and others were reminded of the "cost-savings guarantee."

Planning and Implementation

Another success factor at El Camino was the HCIS's orientation toward "professional" use. Physicians and nurses were to be the key users, rather than clerks and accountants. The product was designed for caregivers' use, but more important, the implementation plan designed by the El Camino staff incorporated physician and nurse involvement at the highest levels and broadly throughout the plan. Physicians, nurses, and other caregivers were system planners, designers, installers, critics, stakeholders, and eventually active users of the HCIS.

The key executive involved in the project—that is, the project champion who possessed the strategic insight and was empowered to move the hospital organization forward by utilizing information technology—was John E. Gall, Jr. Gall, reporting directly to the hospital's administrator, had access to medical staff leaders not only because of the nature of the Lockheed project, but also because of his senior executive status. Frequently, Gall attended hospital board of directors meetings and medical staff committee meetings, and he established solid relationships with key medical staff members.

As the planning of the medical information system (MIS) moved forward, physician involvement became crucial. The widespread participation of the El Camino physicians and the emergence of "medical informatics" champions from their ranks was viewed as contributing significantly to the success of the project. In the earliest planning stages, a few prominent members of the medical staff were asked to participate in critiquing the conceptual model of the MIS. These physicians were selected on the basis of their status in the medical community, their past relationship with the hospital administration and board, and their interest in and comfort with the project. As the conceptual product moved into the pilot test mode, this small group of physicians and surgeons continued its role and became proactive in the design of "their" product. In time, the group expanded to include all medical specialties, and eventually a formal part-time position was created to allow an active volunteer surgeon to be the official leader and liaison for the medical staff with the other information system activists employed by both the vendor/developer and the hospital.

When the MIS migrated from the pilot project to a development effort affecting a larger audience in the hospital, a new constituency of private-practice physicians appeared. Although the earlier controlled group of physicians and surgeons had been invited to be part of the pilot project on the basis of their positive attitudes toward information systems and the hospital itself, the newer, broader-based group did not share the same feelings of loyalty, security, and comfort. In fact, data processing and information technology connoted trouble to many of the private-practice physicians. Their own information system experiences in their private offices were often expensive, with results never living up to expectations. Because most were not computer literate, they had to rely on outside experts to accomplish the simplest computer-related tasks.

Additionally, many of the medical staff members were practicing at El Camino because they enjoyed the uncomplicated environment of the community hospital, which did not offer the complexity of research and teaching programs. The MIS clearly reminded some staff of their previous experiences in training or academic settings.

To counteract this resistance, an intensive effort was undertaken to educate the medical staff at large on the benefits of a clinically focused information system. An equal effort supported correcting the numerous deficiencies identified by the ever-increasing number of physician critics and activists. Of course, some physicians stated up front that they had no interest in the MIS, would not participate in its development, and would never be users, if and when it was implemented. This posture was understood and accepted by those actively involved in the project.

Evaluation

Because El Camino Hospital was not a research or teaching institution and did not have a data processing department and computer equipment on-site, it was by chance that the management staff learned of a potential contract from the Health, Education, and Welfare's National Center for Health Services Research and Development to assess a hospital's information system's impact on the medical, operational, sociological, and economic aspects of health care. Already committed to installing an MIS, the hospital prepared an eleventh-hour proposal to win the contract that would support an analysis of the results of system implementation. Gall became the principal investigator for this important government contract.

The results of the early El Camino project are well documented.[1,2] Much has been written about the benefits derived from utilizing the comprehensive HCIS and its impact on patient care, physician and nurse practice, and hospital operations and economics.

Today, few physicians at El Camino Hospital and the Camino Health-care System are not users of the MIS. The system functions as many of the staff designed it to work, and the high degree of use and satisfaction is directly attributable to the medical staff members' involvement in the project and their obvious status as one of the stakeholders in its success. El Camino Hospital ranks high nationally regarding satisfied physician system users, not only because the medical staff members benefit personally by directly ordering tests and procedures and retrieving results and other information from the computer terminals, but also because they have firsthand knowledge of the positive impact of the information system on their patients, the hospital's nursing staff, and other caregivers and support personnel.

One of the lesser-known, but more interesting, approaches employed at El Camino to establish baseline information for documentation; comparative analysis; and methods, systems, and time studies was El Camino's use of time-lapse photography. Hundreds of rolls of Super-8 movies were shot throughout the hospital to establish a baseline for the delivery of patient care before the implementation of the information system. Admitting areas, medical ancillary reception and waiting locations, all nursing stations, recovery rooms, and other places affected by information system terminals were filmed both before and after implementation. If an eight-second interval was used to study a nursing station, 3,600 "snapshots" (one roll of movie film) were taken on an eight-hour shift. By using a variety of techniques, each of these pictures could accurately measure nursing and physician activity relating to ordering, telephone use, chart review, charting, and so forth. Statistically significant interpretations were made that could be presented in writing or viewed on the movie screen. Time-lapse film analysis allowed change to be described and understood in an easy and comfortable, yet scientific and statistically valid, manner.

El Camino was ahead of its time in the extent of its medical staff's involvement in information system planning and its focus on realizing benefits that allowed the hospital to be more effective and efficient in delivering patient care. More than two decades later, El Camino is still a model hospital and an excellent choice for a site visit; it is one of a small minority of hospitals nationwide that have had significant hospitalwide benefits from information technology. The development of the chief information officer (CIO) role, described in the next section, was another major contribution pioneered at El Camino.

Development of the Chief Information Officer

Until recently, there was little recognition of what it was about the El Camino organizational structure that enabled the project to be successful. Although the formal health care CIO model was not understood in the 1970s, it was Gall who pioneered this role in hospital administration and set an example for a new generation of executives.

Today, the CIO is the senior executive within an organization whose primary responsibility is information management. In collaboration with other senior executives, the CIO is responsible for the development and implementation of the information system strategic plan. Because information is a corporate asset that pervades all areas of an organization, the CIO should be independent and ideally report directly to the CEO.

The CIO works closely with the CEO, senior management, and medical staff on the medical center's strategic goals and integrates the strategic information and technology plan with those goals. With the management team and the Information Systems Steering Committee, the CIO sets the overall architecture, policy, and procedures for information systems in the medical center. The CIO provides the vision and guidance to effectively and creatively influence the use of information technology and the organization's resources for greater organizational effectiveness, as well as the advancement of patient care, education, and research.

The CIO realistically assesses the status of information services at the core components of the medical center and works with their management in determining appropriate directions for the delivery of information and supportive technology. Working with executive management, he or she determines which systems should be centralized and which ones should be decentralized and integrated where appropriate. Further, he or she is the key corporate resource for major hardware and software decisions throughout the medical center. With the steering committee, the CIO has priority-setting and veto authority over all major systems decisions in the medical center.

Characteristics of the CIO position include the ability to fulfill the obligations of a senior executive, in particular, to facilitate the understanding of the other "executive cabinet" members regarding information-related issues. In so doing, the CIO must bridge the gap between the data processing and telecommunications technicians and senior and middle management. Executive management expertise is deemed more important than technological know-how when selecting an appropriate candidate; hence the CIO position is not just a new title for the director of information systems, but an important expansion and increase in responsibilities from technology to management, tactical acting to strategic thinking, reactive work habits to proactive planning, promotion, and marketing.

In 1989, Gall was honored by the Healthcare Information and Management Systems Society (HIMSS) with the society's first CIO Special Recognition Award. Additionally, HIMSS recognized Gall by naming a perpetual CIO award in his honor, which is presented annually to the outstanding health care CIO in the United States and Canada.

Today, a program of the magnitude of the El Camino project should have a formal CIO information management organizational model in place. This ensures the successful implementation of a patient-centered information system among physicians and other users.

Summary

This chapter has provided the rationale for involving physicians in HCISs and has defined what the extent of that involvement really means. The El Camino story provides a historical lesson that is the nucleus of this book's approach to physicians and their use of information systems. The next chapter examines in detail how to plan for and achieve optimum levels of physician involvement, and discusses the perils and pitfalls that are likely to be encountered along the way.

References

1. Gall, J. E., Norwood, D. D., Cook, M., Fleming, J. F., Rydell, R., and Watson, R. J. *Demonstration and Evaluation of a Total Hospital Information System.* NCHSR Research Summary Series. U.S. Department of Health, Education and Welfare Public Health Service, Health Resources Administration, HRA77–3188, July 1977.

2. Gall, J. E., Norwood, D. D., Cook, M., Fleming, J. F., Rydell, R. L., and Watson, R. J. *Demonstration and Evaluation of a Total Hospital Information System.* Mountain View, CA: El Camino Hospital District, Dec. 1975.

Chapter Two

Making a New Beginning: Starting an Information Systems Project

The process of introducing a medical staff to a patient care information system (PCIS) project demands setting a clear vision and expectations for the project. Simply stating that the new project will yield the implementation of a "doctor's system" is sure to engender mistrust from the medical staff and resentment from all other groups working on the project. This chapter focuses on the process of setting a clear vision for medical and enterprise staff and establishing reasonable expectations that will serve the health care organization and its physicians throughout the project.

Finding a Vision and a Common Purpose

At the core of the decision to include physicians in the development of a PCIS is the vision of something better. Apart from the issues of industry trends and pressures, such as providing cost-of-care information mentioned in chapter 1, there needs to be the vision among the health care administration that incorporating physicians into the selection, definition, and implementation of a PCIS is the *right* thing to do. This vision must be grounded in an understanding of the history of the health care organization; the needs of the community it serves; the institution's culture, goals, and values; and the groups that will need to be involved to reach the desired end point. Furthermore, although this vision is rather obvious once it is under serious consideration, it can be formulated only when everyone serving the hospital puts aside his or her fear of change.

The origin of a vision to involve physicians in information system development may be found at any level of the organization and in either the administrative or clinical realm. It is often surprising to health care organization supporters how powerful a vision of this sort can be and how readily it can spread throughout the enterprise. However, there are those who are against its dissemination.

In the current era of special-interest groups and lobbies, it is sometimes difficult to identify the common goal or purpose that bring us together as a country. Sometimes, as in the recent Desert Storm conflict, these common goals are recognized and affirmed, and patriotism flourishes. However, more often we are faced with the competing agendas of many special-interest groups, as in the common national financial crises of trade deficit and recession.

Extending these observations to the health care field is both easy and appropriate. The United States' current state of having both the most technically advanced and the most inaccessible and expensive health care system in the world is testimony to health care's lack of common purpose. External costs and regulatory pressures make it all too easy for the gulf between health care administrations and medical staffs to widen.

It is the uncommon administrator and clinician who realize that these trends will do nothing but erode the quality of patient care and even collapse the health care system altogether. These champions of the common purposes of health care—that is, service and patient care—are the persons most likely to originate the vision of administration and physicians collaboratively pursuing a new PCIS. When these champions can overcome the *common wisdom* of special-interest organizational politics, the process can then begin to develop a PCIS that is responsive to the needs of physicians.

Making It Personal: Identifying the Champions

The beginning of a PCIS project may take many forms: a review of previous information system plans, a realization that the institution needs a system, the medical staff's request for easier access to care for their patients, and so forth. Regardless of the source of the PCIS vision, champions of the system must be identified at the outset of the project to begin to propagate the concepts of information system design, as well as its expected benefits, among all potential user groups. Although some talented individuals can assume both the administrator's and the clinician's role as champion, most often representatives from both spheres must be identified or cultivated. Persons from different levels of the administration and medical staff may fill this responsibility; however, specific *profiles for success* in both the administrator champion and the physician champion can be identified as follows.

The administrator champion should function at or near the highest possible level of senior management. His or her perspective should include the current and future needs of the institution and the community it serves. Specific computer-related expertise is far less important than the ability to see the 5- to 10-year plan of the institution and to have access to senior management to make this plan a reality. At various institutions, this administrator champion has been a CIO, a CEO, a chief operating officer (COO), a chief financial officer (CFO), or an information systems department director, among others. Specific experience in communicating with the medical staff is helpful. More important, however, is the willingness to reach out and bridge the gap between administration and medical staff.

To be effective, the physician champion must be well recognized and respected by the medical staff. A working knowledge of the formal and informal leadership of the medical staff is essential to successfully bring the PCIS vision to the staff and enlist buy-in and support. Having recognition for clinical expertise is far more important in this regard than having a reputation as a "gadgeteer."

Furthermore, the physician champion should be a champion for the common purposes of service and patient care among all caregivers, as well as for the development of the PCIS. That is, he or she should understand the needs of the nursing staff, physicians, and support services staff. For example, a clear understanding of precisely how medication orders are processed in the hospital will lead to the conclusion that physicians must directly enter orders into an information system for greatest efficiency, which will directly benefit patients, pharmacy, and nursing. Conversely, details of discharge planning may be best left to a specialized nursing service advising the attending physician. Even if the physician champion has been in practice for many years, additional education will be necessary to allow him or her to understand the interrelationships among health care personnel and how the information system should operate and be used to best support high-quality patient care.

Although the foregoing has implied a single physician champion, there are other workable approaches, including the establishment of a physician steering committee. A panel of physician champions would minimize the strain of time commitment on the part of any one member and also could provide a broader representation of the staff than any one individual. On the downside, this model could also diffuse responsibility and potentially complicate communication.

Regardless of the structure, the sooner a physician champion or group of champions is recognized, the better it is for the project. Physician champions are one of the most powerful sources of trust among the medical staff.

The formalized commitment between the administration and the physician champion and the timing of this agreement also are important. There is little doubt that the time commitment to the PCIS project by the physician champion will be significant. The responsibilities of system selection, coordination of the process of the design of the physician's portion of the PCIS, and participation in physician education and implementation are significant and time-consuming. One method of coping with this is to offer the physician champion a formal part-time position in the administrative structure of the health care organization. This commitment signals the first significant change in attitude on the part of both the medical staff and the administration. It is essential that the clinician not completely abandon his or her practice to serve the PCIS project, because a continued clinical perspective and visibility among other physicians are essential for his or her effectiveness as the physician champion of the project. Figure 2-1 provides an example of a contract between a physician and a hospital for his or her service as a PCIS champion.

Early recruitment of the physician champion into the PCIS project is one of the most powerful means of communicating a commitment to involve the medical staff. The story of the information system rejected by the medical staff when physicians perceived that they were the last ones notified is almost a proverb. Proactive assignment of a PCIS medical director signals a new relationship between administration and physicians that will serve well during the later stresses of system configuration and implementation.

Three elements ensure a strong collaborative relationship between the physician champion and the CIO or administrative champions: cooperation, trust, and team building and infrastructure.

Cooperation refers to a mutual understanding of a physician's attitudes and motivations in order to begin a relationship. The factors to consider are the physician's role as patient advocate; his or her demand for greater efficiency, a demand that stems from current financial and regulatory pressures

Figure 2-1. Sample Contract for a PCIS Champion

Dr. _____ will be responsible to the Vice-President of Information Systems, St. Elsewhere Hospital. He/she is responsible for the development, utilization, and integration of clinical information systems throughout St. Elsewhere. This includes, but is not limited to:

  a. Integrating the clinical information systems, including but not limited to the nursing information office, the laboratories, radiology, pharmacy, and the ancillary services information office
  b. Determining medical staff and house staff needs for clinical information systems
  c. Developing compatible clinical information systems for all of St. Elsewhere's subsidiaries, including strategic planning
  d. Establishing clinical information systems objectives consonant with the goals and major policy directions of the clinical services at St. Elsewhere and other subsidiaries that will result in systems that contribute to the achievement of higher-quality patient care
  e. Collaborating with clinical departments to identify significant clinical needs and developing working information systems that will meet those needs
  f. Providing leadership in the development of policy, practices, and procedures governing clinical information systems, clinical data processing operations, and the management of medical information system facilities

Should Dr. _____'s time commitment exceed 000 hours per year (that is, 0.0 FTE) during the term of the Agreement, the physician reserves the right to renegotiate the Agreement accordingly.

on clinical practice; and the history at the particular institution of the relationship between the administration and the medical staff. To illustrate this last factor, take time to reflect on the following question: How would the members of your hospital's medical staff characterize the attitude of the hospital administration: facilitating? indifferent? obstructionist? The answer may provide a clue as to the kind of support your physician champion will need in order to make the PCIS project successful.

Trust refers to a physician's better understanding of the work of health care administrators and, in particular, information system administrators. An essential factor in building trust is the education of the physician champion and medical staff, for this is truly unknown territory for the average clinician. However, it should be cautioned that overemphasis of the technology and distinct language of information systems only further alienates a medical staff. The more the information system operations can be described in clinical and common terms, the better it is for building trust with the physician champion. An additional factor in building trust is the degree to which the information systems director can enlist other allies to communicate with the physician champion and medical staff. Often office managers and nurses can act as facilitators for physicians to better understand the information systems operation and foster the trust between physicians and the information systems administration.

Team building and infrastructure refer to the creation of established task force structures that foster effective communication between the information systems administration and the physician champion and medical staff. The composition, operation, and support of the long-term physician committee structure is crucial to the productivity and strength of the information systems administration–physician champion relationship. In a later section, this chapter discusses the creation and selection of a physician task force.

Introducing the Vision to the Medical Staff: The PCIS Imperative

The first task in engaging the medical staff in the PCIS vision is the education of the physician champion. In light of the aforementioned selection criteria, this physician will not likely have a strong background in HCISs. Site visits and conferences should be employed to increase the physician's knowledge of PCISs.

Although site visits are a popular means of gaining specific knowledge of information systems, they often are costly mistakes. Thorough knowledge of the specific strengths and weaknesses of system implementations, as well as of the key individuals to meet, is essential to obtaining maximum benefit from the experience. All too often, a potential PCIS system is rejected because of a chance visit to a below-average installation. It is essential to purposefully select sites that will help answer questions relevant to one's own PCIS and institution. Consider the following checklist when evaluating sites:

1. Is this institution similar to your own in size, demographics, structure of medical staff (open/closed), and training programs?
2. To what extent do physicians really use the information system at this institution? (See the definitions of the levels of involvement in chapter 1.)
3. What departments have most successfully implemented the PCIS at this site?
4. Do the departments that have been unsuccessful provide an important object lesson that needs to be communicated to your health care organization (for example, lack of early involvement of staff, failure to customize the information tools to fit the users, poor management of change in the department, and so forth)?
5. Are the directors of the PCIS at this site willing to customize the tour to meet your needs, including arranging specific interviews with physician users?

Without a careful screening of sites for the specific information and experience the organization is looking for, a site visit can be simply an expensive fishing expedition. Choose wisely!

Following the education of the physician champion, it is time to begin transferring that individual's enthusiasm and knowledge to his or her physician colleagues, that is, to begin initiating the medical staff into the information systems project. These introductory days also further establish the physician champion as the system's advocate and *local expert* in the eyes of the medical staff. Although styles, forums, and content will be different in each health care organization's situation, there are several themes that need to be presented to the medical staff to maximize the project's potential for success.

First, bring home the patient care imperative. The common denominators of the medical staff are their concern for patient care and their recognized position as patient advocates. The PCIS must be described and recognized as promoting the physician's role as director of the health care process and must demonstrate clear benefits that will result in improvement in the quality of patient care. Patient advocacy is one of the *hot buttons* for all physicians. If every opportunity is made to introduce the PCIS as affecting and enhancing the advocacy role, physician attention will follow. Conversely, if technology and change are the messages, a much smaller proportion of the staff will stand up and take notice.

Second, emphasize the communication aspects of the PCIS as also supporting the demands of clinical practice. The life of most clinicians today is characterized by trying to do more and more in less and less time. The regulatory and reimbursement themes of health care are taking a toll on every practice, so a tool that promises relief from the inefficiencies of the office–hospital link will be most welcome. Although this theme may be described only in the context of in-hospital practice, its most powerful extension is the potential for extending PCIS access to physician offices (see chapter 5).

Third, address the two earliest concerns that physicians have when beginning to understand a PCIS: access and security. Concern over access to the PCIS arises from most clinicians' inability to translate the way they use a paper record to the way they would use the new electronic record. Obviously, the extent of this translation will depend on the functionality of your system, that is, whether it offers complete order entry and results reporting or just the generation of the physician's patient lists. Here, the physician champion's site visit experience can hold sway with reluctant physicians by indicating that in the real world, physicians can and do carry out rounds with a finite number of terminals per nursing unit. More important, this is the opportunity to inform the medical staff that the hospital's implementation of a PCIS will include a mechanism to ensure physician access and terminal use that will be carefully monitored and adjusted to ensure service and responsiveness.

Although PCIS security is discussed fully in chapter 6, it deserves a mention at this point. Even at this early phase in the medical staff's understanding of the PCIS, it is important to manage the information regarding system security. To begin, security must be differentiated from confidentiality. *Security* relates to the ability of the system to maintain the integrity of the patient's electronic record, to provide some manner of password restriction of access to that electronic record, and to be reliable in presenting the record. In contrast, *confidentiality* relates only to the restrictions on use of patient care information by the potential users of the PCIS. At this stage in the project, the medical staff should understand that the PCIS has adequate and effective security safeguards but that in no way will these replace the need for effective confidentiality policies and practices. Most important, a PCIS security committee should be formed early in the project, with physician representation, to provide the health care organization with a process for handling all its concerns about security and confidentiality as they arise.

Fourth, describe the PCIS to the medical staff as a clinical information tool rather than a technological wonder. Unfortunately, our culture has already generated the term *computer literacy,* which tends to alienate persons who are outside the computing inner circle. This alienation, and the fear it causes, has likely already touched many of the medical staff physicians who watch their children working on personal computers (PCs) at home. The physician champion strategy, which serves to maintain an emphasis on the clinical tool fitting the needs of physician users, is key to avoiding any further promotion of this sense of alienation and the resistance born of fear. Obviously, the test of these concerns will finally occur when the first terminal is available for physician review. However, at this early stage sensitivity to the physicians' insecurity regarding this perceived foreign realm is essential. Expressing this project's commitment to direct clinical usability of the PCIS will pay dividends in acceptance throughout the life of the project.

Fifth, build a foundation of trust between the medical staff and the administration. That sentence is easy to write but difficult to accomplish! The success of the collaboration between the clinical staff and the administration with regard to the implementation of a comprehensive PCIS will depend on the strength of the relationship between the administrative champion and the physician champion. Clearly, this is where the attention of the medical staff should initially be focused to demonstrate that the PCIS project is not "business as usual."

Sixth, be sensitive to intra–medical-staff conflicts that may surface during the changes brought on by the introduction of the PCIS. Many institutions have a medical staff split between hospital-based physicians and community-based physicians. If the medical staff has a history of strong subgroups such as these, specific issues that are of greatest interest to each group will need to be evaluated and addressed. For example, community physicians may be most keenly interested in the integration of their office practice with the hospital's PCIS, whereas hospital staff physicians may be most interested in using the new information system for clinical research and education. Representatives from each group must be included in PCIS planning or valuable perspectives will be lost.

This so-called *town–gown* distinction must be recognized and incorporated into the medical staff's introduction to the PCIS and in the composition of PCIS physician task forces. Most important, avoid the myth of medical staff consensus. How many issues has your medical staff resolved with greater than 80 percent agreement? The 80/20 rule of decision making, that is, the test of acceptability is positive if it serves physicians 80 percent of the time, should be the guide for medical staff consensus.

Seventh, recognize actual practice patterns in describing the manner in which the PCIS will be useful clinically. For example, a university hospital in which residents perform 90 percent (or more) of actual patient orders and a small community hospital in which 100 percent of orders come from primary care physicians pose two very different challenges to PCIS design and introduction. In the former situation, the design of PCIS pathways would be directed by the residents and medical education would be part of the system's design. In the latter situation, primary emphasis would be placed on the speed with which the system could be used, customizing system design so that each physician group would see its own list of common medications, laboratory tests, radiology examinations, and so on. Obviously, the ultimate efficiency would be an information system that has the ability to be customized by the individual. Because an individual physician's needs are best known to that person alone, and because the needs of the individual practitioner change over time, the best strategy is the development of easy-to-use tools for user customization of the PCIS.

Eighth, emphasize that the medical staff's opinions and participation are being sought *from the outset* in this PCIS project. At one level this strategy reinforces the respect and relationship between administration and medical staff. More important, however, it signals the creation of a working partnership, most evidently symbolized by the administrator and physician champions, to achieve the goal of improving the quality of patient care.

Ninth, consider administering a physician PCIS survey. In some settings a questionnaire polling opinions, needs, and concerns may be useful following the initial presentation of the PCIS project to the medical staff. Be aware, however, that most physicians receive a great many of these questionnaires and quickly direct most of them to the "circular file." Alternatively, a question-and-answer session during group staff meetings can be used to achieve the same purpose. An example of a medical staff questionnaire is shown in figure 2-2.

Finally, build on the fact that everybody loves a winner. Distinguish the health care organization's efforts at selecting and implementing a PCIS as special right from the start. Internal marketing and publicity should receive attention from the start to encourage the medical staff's confidence in both the process and the physician champion. For example, frequent presentations

Figure 2-2.   Sample Physician PCIS Survey

1. Do you currently use computers in your practice?
2. If yes, how are they used?
3. If not, are you planning to computerize? When?
4. If your answer to the first question was yes, what is your opinion of the usefulness of computers in your practice?
5. How do you think computers could help in your personal practice requirements?
6. The hospital would like your input in the selection of a new patient care information system. Would you be interested in participating in a physician task force to work on the project?
7. What features of a patient care information system would be most important to you?
8. Would you be interested in an office computer linkage with this patient care information system?
9. Where should terminals be placed in the hospital to make the patient care information system most accessible for you?
10. What issues should be addressed to make you personally more comfortable in using a patient care information system?

on the system at medical staff and departmental meetings or demonstrations of the system (staffed or stand-alone) in the physician lounge areas are means of keeping the project current for the medical staff. Often the most effective early publicity for internal consumption arises from an external source. That is, consider holding early grand rounds on PCISs by a recognized expert in the field (preferably a physician who can speak firsthand to both the clinical and the technological virtues of PCISs). Such a presentation, which might conclude with special recognition of the hospital's efforts, can be a powerful milestone launching the medical staff's involvement in the process.

Developing the Infrastructure: The Physician Task Force

After a general introduction of the PCIS to the medical staff, it is time to organize a physician task force. The physician champion should select and lead this body throughout the PCIS project, including system selection, configuration, and implementation.

The charges of this task force should include:

- To represent the needs and interests of the medical staff in the selection, design, testing, and implementation of the PCIS
- To communicate issues back to the staff at large
- To develop the policies and procedures necessary to facilitate use of the PCIS by the medical staff
- To recognize opportunities to change current practices and policies to take better advantage of the PCIS in order to improve the quality and efficiency of care delivery
- To act as advocates for the PCIS

System selection, design, and implementation are dealt with in chapter 4. Task force selection, meeting design, and the communication network deserve special mention here.

Selecting the Physician Task Force

Selection of the physician task force is one activity that is crucial to the success of the PCIS project. Criteria for inclusion in this seven- or eight-member group should include:

- Substantial influence with clinicians. Physicians who consistently influence the practice patterns of their peers and are well respected for their medical acumen are the true movers and shakers of the medical staff, although they may or may not be formal heads of divisions. If the physician champion comes from the ranks of active medical staff, these individuals will not be difficult for him or her to identify; however, a simple, informal poll of staff members will also help identify these outstanding individuals. Unfortunately, these individuals often are the busiest clinically, with little time to spend at meetings. It is a challenge to the physician champion to persuade these individuals that their participation in the PCIS project is crucial to the clinical value of the system.

- Representation from all major clinical divisions (for example, medicine, surgery, pediatrics, and so forth). However, in the aforementioned town–gown situations, both in-hospital and community physicians need to be adequately represented on the team.
- Commitment to making the health care organization a better place for patient care. Despite their demanding schedules, clinically influential physicians must be willing to contribute time and effort to the PCIS project and be supportive of the final goal. The task force's job will likely be a long and hard one, and obviously one or two obstructive, divisive members can markedly impair the productivity of the group.
- Some degree of interest in the technology and a willingness to learn. This is not to suggest that members must be technophiles — far from it. Emphasis must be on the fact that clinically competent physicians do not have to be elitist computer experts to learn and use the PCIS.
- A good working knowledge of the existing review and approval committee structure in the institution. This is desirable, although not essential. The volume of information, interrelationships, and changes engendered by the PCIS creates abundant opportunities to affect current policies and practices. A physician with a good sense of the best path through the maze can be an invaluable facilitator and help avoid conflict between proposed PCIS operation and organizational policy.

Designing and Conducting Meetings

Meeting design and conduct are likewise crucial to the success of the physician task force. The following considerations clearly fall more in the realm of art than of science, but through experience have proved helpful.

Meeting Time and Place

Task force meetings for physicians with busy clinical practices should be limited to twice monthly. If the organization of the meetings is effective in maximizing productivity, the rest of the PCIS development team will require the 15-day interval to respond to the task force's recommendations and reviews. Meeting time should be chosen to minimize interruptions from pocket beepers, which usually means planning the meeting for either early morning or late afternoon. The surgical members of the group usually have the most difficult schedules, and working around their availability is often the rule. As early as possible in the process, a dedicated PCIS room should be identified. Terminals linked with the test systems should be available simply to focus members' attention on the reality and immediacy of their project and to provide hands-on opportunities.

Meeting Design

Attention to preparation is essential to obtain maximum performance from the physician task force. Routine preparation of required reading material mailed one to two weeks prior to meetings can double the effectiveness and productivity of meetings. Reading material includes:

- Articles published in the medical literature on computers in medicine (*Journal of the American Medical Association* and the *Annals of Internal Medicine* are two particularly good resources)
- Abstracts of current clinical policies that will need to be amended to take advantage of the new information system
- Printouts of examples of system form and content (that is, screen display printouts)

As a rule, physicians will prefer to render opinions over a range of clearly presented choices. Whenever possible, try to demonstrate several options for the group's review rather than creating de novo. Remember, this group was chosen on the basis of its members' clinical acumen, not their computer expertise. If the level of discussion is consistently pitched at clinical relevance and patient care issues, members will be more apt to participate and more comfortable with their role.

The technique of asking for special reports by ad hoc subgroups of the main task force provides another opportunity to expand the group's overall productivity as well as increase the ownership of, and commitment to, the process by the task force physicians. Consider asking a support person to attend the meeting to take minutes; it can be quite a chore to keep track of all the ideas and decisions once this group really starts to get down to business. The imperative to document all activities arises from the magnitude and duration of the project. Remember, old issues never die, they just come back to haunt you!

Building the Communication Network

Attention should also be paid to the communication network between the physician task force and key groups within the health care organization. Four main groups should be addressed:

1. PCIS steering committee (senior executives and physicians and ancillary department directors acting in an oversight capacity)
2. The PCIS management group within the information systems department
3. The medical staff
4. Health care organization operational committees

The physician champion should act as the link between the physician task force and the PCIS management group, that is, the group within the information systems department that is doing the actual planning of the PCIS. Minutes of the physician task force meetings should be distributed to this PCIS management group as well.

Communication with the medical staff should be designed to serve several goals:

- To progressively educate the medical staff as to what the PCIS is and the impact it will have on staff members
- To facilitate departmental dialogue among physicians to plan for the PCIS
- To process *special issues* such as system security and confidentiality and, as much as possible, to make use of existing medical staff committee structures to complement the work of the PCIS security committee

Mechanisms to achieve these goals include monthly physician bulletins and presentations to staff and at departmental meetings.

Wherever possible, the physician task force should use the existing communication network for organizational operations. Changes in policy and procedures are common during the configuration and implementation of a PCIS. More efficient use of time and better communication are both served by using standing operational committee structures.

Nevertheless, it is essential to identify when decisions need to be made outside the physician task force and when they need to be made by the task force itself. As a rule of thumb, if a decision relates to the best way to design, operate, or use the PCIS, more than likely the physician task force is empowered to make this judgment. If, on the other hand, a decision changes basic operating policies and procedures to make best use of the PCIS, the issue should be processed through the existing health care organization's committee structure.

For example, consider the following scenario: The physician task force is presented with several alternative ways of retrieving patient laboratory and department results on-line. In this situation, the task force physicians are the topic experts and should make the decision.

Now consider this scenario: On-line drug ordering now makes it possible to set up a physician reminder system that brings different classes of drugs up for renewal at specific intervals (for example, seven days for antibiotics, three days for narcotics, and so on). In this situation, the existing hospital pharmacy committee's input should be solicited. This usually will expedite a decision, communicate the change to all necessary parties, and further educate professionals outside the task force regarding the nature of the PCIS.

In addition, certain issues require a degree of validation from outside bodies. For example, a resolution to abandon written order sheets as the standard method of physician ordering may evolve in the physician task force. However, it would be folly not to validate this opinion with the medical staff governing bodies. When this validation occurs, a strong message is sent to the administration, as well as all other groups in the institution, that the medical staff is strongly behind the PCIS effort.

Summary

This chapter has presented approaches to involving physicians in the PCIS project, including techniques and organizational structures. However, with a project of the magnitude of an enterprisewide information system, planning cannot anticipate all the potential problems and roadblocks. The next chapter reviews approaches to the constellation of problems that often present themselves when trying to obtain physician involvement in a PCIS project.

Trials and Tribulations: What to Do When Things Do Not Go Well

The troubles that can plague the best-planned projects are discussed in this chapter. Problems related to software selection or performance will be addressed separately in chapter 4. This chapter begins by identifying the key groups that can adversely affect physician utilization of a PCIS. They are:

- Physicians
- Information systems or data processing personnel
- Executive management (administrators)

The final portion of this chapter discusses special problem situations.

Barriers from Physicians

The most successful group at derailing physician acceptance and use of a PCIS is the medical staff itself. There are as many different responses and reactions to the PCIS among members of the medical staff as there are different personalities. However, these destructive responses can be summarized in several categories:

- Reaction to change
- The fallacy of computer literacy
- Deferral of responsibility
- Computerphobia and computermania

Reaction to Change

Change is a given in our present-day environment, and health care is one area that has provided some of the most challenging patterns of change over the past 10 years. Individual responses to change cover the spectrum from fear and avoidance to cautious evaluation and consideration, to aggressive acceptance and motivation, and finally to more change. Physician response to change likewise covers this gamut, but tends to be weighted toward the more conservative end of the spectrum — fear and avoidance — and for good reasons. Physicians are at the top of the clinical chain of command and occupy the most visible, vulnerable position of authority and accountability. The paranoia and "defensive medicine" trends apparent among today's clinicians bear witness to this. Therefore, conservatism has arisen in response to the tremendous external changes that have affected physicians over the past 10 years.

Because the health care system has largely been affected by outside agencies, the primary concern among physicians is that they have lost control of the situation. If it is not promoted and handled with this fact in mind, the introduction of a hospital PCIS can appear as simply the latest example of the physicians' loss of control. The most effective antidote to this reaction to change is the appointment of the physician champion. If properly promoted, this individual will be perceived as the *insider* looking out for the concerns and interests of the medical staff. Regular communication with the medical staff will reinforce this perception.

It is important to differentiate the medical staff's legitimate conservative reaction to change from its more extreme reaction of obstructionist behavior. The unyielding resistance to any alteration in "business as usual" may be manifested by a few individuals, usually those with a history of similar behavior. If not dealt with properly, these individuals can impede the progress of a PCIS project.

The most effective means of dealing with this minority of unyielding physicians is peer pressure. Through peer pressure, the majority of physician staff members who recognize that change is inevitable can slowly but surely override the unrealistic, obstructive voices on the staff. The tactic of obtaining a medical staff resolution in support of the PCIS early in the process may also be an effective way to signal medical staff dissidents that there is in fact general support to move ahead. For example, the executive council of the medical staff of Baystate Medical Center in Springfield, Massachusetts, adopted a resolution that stated in part:

> The Medical Staff hereby resolves that 12 months following the completion of Phase II of the implementation of the Patient Care Information System, the standard method of physician ordering will be through direct-order entry into this patient care communication system. Written orders will be acceptable only as a backup during system downtime.
>
> Physician training will be ensured by physician-directed, small-group training sessions and personal one-on-one training.

The Fallacy of Computer Literacy

One of the most unfortunate terms in modern parlance is *computer literacy.* In the context of destructive responses to physician involvement in a PCIS, this term has been used in two ways:

1. As an elitist slogan
2. As an excuse for passive abdication of involvement and understanding by the medical staff

Computer literacy as an elitist slogan is proposed by the technocrats of the medical staff or data processing department to set up an "us versus them" situation with the rest of the medical staff. This phrase is used to explain everything from why physicians are unable to comprehend and use an arcane information system to why the staff is uninterested in long technical explanations of system operation. This situation is patently destructive to the process of physician involvement in a PCIS and often evokes an angry response from the victim. The best way to counteract the use of this destructive term is to promote the service aspect of the PCIS project. *Service* means that the most important responsibility of the PCIS team is to make the technology understandable and usable for the medical staff and, further, to have the information tool fit the user.

Lack of computer literacy is sometimes used as an excuse by members of the medical staff to abdicate their responsibility for learning to use a PCIS. The arguments usually go something like this: "I'm too old to learn this stuff." Or, "This will work only with the new residents, who have had all this in medical school." Or even, "I've got one of these at home and my kid uses it, but I'm totally clueless."

This passive, dependent behavior is more difficult to deal with, but it can be rectified. The passive but receptive individual will begin to respond to individual attention and instruction. In addition, certain aspects of system design will have a profound effect on breaking down some of these barriers of understanding. For example, physicians are interested in pathways for ordering that connect clinically valid information, such as displaying the orders for Coumadin and prothrombin at the same time on the same screen.

However, some individuals will inevitably continue to use their lack of computer literacy as a barrier. When attempts are made to educate them, they may respond with anger and the aforementioned obstructionism. Again, peer pressure is the most effective mechanism in this case to wear down resistance over time.

Deferral of Responsibility

Deferral of responsibility is one of the most insidious and difficult barriers to deal with. For example, a physician may offer to cooperate in using the system by "having my secretary [or intern, nurse, and so on] learn how to use this thing." This reaction is a natural one for the busy clinician. A physician with an active practice is accustomed to having his or her staff interact with many different technologies, including computers. In particular, assigning staff members to interact with computers seems natural to some physicians because the computer's similarity to a typewriter often gives the impression that it is more a clerical device than a patient management tool.

The best way to counteract this barrier is through physician education and the demonstration of practice benefits. The educator must change the perception of the computer from a clerical tool to a patient care tool. Once the power and importance of controlling this new tool is made manifest to the physician, the deferral of responsibility problem usually abates. Physicians do not defer responsibility for using the stethoscope, a trusted tool, to other persons. Similarly, they must entrust the use of the PCIS with the same regard.

Computerphobia and Computermania

At one end of the technology spectrum is the physician with computerphobia; at the other end is the physician with computermania. Both maladaptations can be destructive to the overall process of physician involvement in a PCIS project. Fortunately, physicians with either of these extreme orientations are in the minority on most medical staffs, comprising less than 25 percent of the total membership. Computerphobes without additional agendas can usually be approached in a one-on-one, physician-to-physician manner with some success. Nurse–physician *buddy-system* arrangements can also be effective in some instances and can even promote more effective PCIS use by noncomputerphobe physicians.

Computermaniacs, or *techies,* are becoming more and more common and are more difficult to deal with. These physicians have been exposed to the microcomputing world and often own one or more computers. They are enthusiastic and typically want to be among the first clinicians to join the physician task force. However, their love of computers often is coupled with a myopia regarding the magnitude of the computing challenge of automating an entire health care enterprise. All too often, the computer-enthusiast physician is the first one to become impatient with a system that superficially seems no more complicated than his or her PC database manager. This impatience and lack of perspective can be disconcerting to other physicians, because they can change the focus of discussions from whether the PCIS will work effectively to improve the quality of patient care to whether the PCIS is state of the art.

Modern PCISs are offering more and more features that interest the physician techie. Therefore, one method of using these physicians to best advantage is to assign them to an advanced computer development subgroup of the physician task force, which often can lead to a productive relationship. Another effective method for minimizing the influence of the computermaniac is to continually reinforce the clinical aspects of the PCIS implementation during meetings with physicians. The majority of the clinicians will be more comfortable in such discussions, and the techies will have less time to dwell on the arcane.

Barriers from Information Systems or Data Processing Personnel

Problems with physician involvement in the PCIS may also be presented by information systems or data processing personnel. Data processing personnel often talk about "controlling" physician input into PCIS design and implementation, and they often profile physicians as "too demanding" of their time and effort. Unfortunately, some data processing departments have developed without the service paradigm; that is, they fail to recognize that the efforts of all the members of an institution must be directed to the support and aid of the common goals of that institution and the people carrying out those goals. In health care organizations, the common goal is patient care. The people carrying out that goal are physicians, nurses, and other health care workers. Regrettably, some information systems departments have evolved as self-important and seemingly self-contained entities without a pervasive sense of service to the institution or of the department's role within the institution. It is easy to see from this insulated perspective how information systems departments could react negatively to complaints from physicians and then actively seek to exclude physicians from decision making and involvement in the PCIS.

The most effective antidotes to this barrier are peer pressure and the evolution of greater administrative demands on the information system. Fortunately, the same forces that have led to an increased interest in PCISs among administrators—financial constraints, increased regulatory standards, quality assurance—have also led to increased demands that measurable clinical benefits be obtained as a result of installing a PCIS. As the clinical benefits of PCISs become more commonly recognized, more health care leaders will demand this kind of return on their PCIS investment from the information systems management team.

National information systems organizations, such as the Healthcare Information and Management Systems Society and the College of Healthcare Information Management Executives (CHIME), are now actively promoting clinician involvement in PCIS programs as one of the keys to the success of these systems. In addition, the common pressures of tighter regulations and financial controls on hospitals force information systems departments to get the most from their information investments, stimulating a reaching out to clinical staff to ensure that new systems will be accepted and used successfully.

Barriers from Executive Management (Administrators)

Health care administrators also can fail to adopt the service paradigm and can develop several destructive reactions that block physician involvement in a PCIS. Three common negative responses are:

- "The administration cannot afford physician involvement."
- "Physician desires are incompatible with the desires of the health care organization."
- "Physicians are too difficult to work with."

"The Administration Cannot Afford Physician Involvement"

There are three possible reasons for an administrator's statement that physician involvement cannot be afforded:

1. Administrators are afraid that if physicians become involved with the PCIS, administrators will not be able to control the physicians' interest and zeal to do more and more.
2. Administrators do not trust the medical staff to work in the best interests of the health care organization, and fear that physician agendas will overextend the time and money budget.
3. Administrators do not like working with physicians in general.

Thus, under the guise of financial concerns, many messages are being communicated about the relationship between a mistrustful hospital administration and the hospital's medical staff. To some extent, the trends of national health care executive groups and peer pressure are beginning to reveal that mistrustful behavior is unacceptable and counterproductive in the health care enterprise of the 1990s. However, in some cases the history of the institution and poor communication between administrators and physicians are the fuels that keep these fires of destruction burning. If a physician champion can be selected and supported, part of his or her role will be to bridge this gulf and educate both the administration *and* the medical staff so that these two factions can work together productively on a project of the magnitude of a PCIS.

"Physician Desires Are Incompatible with the Desires of the Health Care Organization"

As has already been discussed, the administration's response to physician involvement in a PCIS may be related to poor communication. It can also be related to poor selection of physician representatives. Occasionally, the wrong message is sent to the administration by unrepresentative members of the medical staff. For example, physician computerphobe or computermaniac minority voices can sometimes become the most strident when administration begins to evaluate medical staff interest in a PCIS. This issue underscores the importance of careful selection of a physician champion for the project. One of the physician champion's most important roles is to correctly tap the majority opinion on the medical staff regarding a PCIS and deal appropriately with the extremes.

"Physicians Are Too Difficult to Work With"

Whether explicit or implicit, the statement that administrators find physicians difficult to work with is destructive and capable of completely derailing efforts at involving the medical staff in a PCIS project. The problem here is that the statement has an element of truth to it. Physicians are by nature individualists, opinionated, and impatient for progress, especially when it relates to improving the quality of care for their patients and making their practice lives more efficient and effective.

In large measure, the careful and complete education of the administration and the medical staff regarding the complexity of the PCIS and its implementation can counteract this maladaptive reaction. Again, communication is the key: The structures for physician representation in the project and feedback from the physician task force to the administration should be planned out carefully, with clearly assigned individuals making the information links work.

Special Cases

Finally, there are some special situations that can significantly affect the goal of physician involvement in a PCIS. These may be termed: the second time around, the last straw, and the vocal minority.

The Second Time Around

One of the most difficult challenges facing some health care organizations is to revive medical staff interest in an information system that has been in place for some time without significant usage by physicians. Assuming that the installed system does in fact have functionality that is useful to clinicians, this unfortunate situation presents several roadblocks:

1. Unfavorable patterns of physician interaction with the information system are already established.
2. Physician opinion is that the medical staff was specifically excluded from planning the system.
3. System development decisions (regarding terminal access and system operation, for example) were made without consideration of direct clinician use.

The third issue is better dealt with in chapter 4 in the discussion of system design necessary to support clinician use. The first two issues deserve further explanation here.

Dealing with Established Patterns of Physician Usage

As mentioned earlier in this chapter, one of the most difficult problems physicians present to the use of information tools is deferral of responsibility. For health care organizations wishing to involve physicians in established information systems, this deferral is fully operative. Busy clinicians have already completely adapted to the information system, and perhaps even effectively so, by having their staff members access the system for them. In consideration of the physician's role within the clinical team, a reversal of responsibilities to engage the PCIS usually brings outrage that the physician "now has to do the nurse's, intern's, or secretary's work!" Furthermore, the initial learning curve that would be present for physicians for any PCIS is even less palatable because of established patterns of practice.

The most effective way to counteract these problems is to reintroduce the PCIS. Simply put, the PCIS must be reviewed, repackaged, enhanced, and "re-presented" to the medical staff as an entirely new tool intended for their direct use. Obviously, this effort would be identified as a sham if important changes and enhancements were not in fact being planned. However, in a setting where the information system has been developed without physician input, there are usually numerous aspects of its operation that would need to be reviewed and renovated, which would justify the reintroduction.

The addition of *entirely new* technology to such a system is ideal, but not totally necessary. For example, the information system might be introduced into the physicians' offices to signal the medical staff that something new really is happening. By the nature of this move, modifications to the PCIS would be required to make it useful in the physician office setting. Although the extent of the planning requirements and task force responsibilities for such a modification is not as great as that required for an entirely new PCIS installation, a task force and planning structure should nevertheless be created to send clear signals to the entire health care organization and medical staff that new effort and vigor is being applied to physician involvement in information tools. This approach will produce results that can be identical to the introduction of an entirely new system.

Dealing with Physicians Who Have Felt Excluded from Planning

Poor communication is the most common reason for the perception that physicians were excluded from previous PCIS plans. However, for all intents and purposes, perception is fact, and a good deal of effort must be expended to enhance communication in order to erase this past impression. The ways to reverse this perception include:

- The selection and empowerment of a physician PCIS champion
- Staff meeting presentations with regular updates

- Special written communications reflecting how physician input has changed the design and implementation of the new PCIS program

The Last Straw

A second special case affecting the extent of physician acceptance of information tools may be termed *the last straw*. When a health care organization and its medical staff have been at odds for some time because of poor communication and misunderstanding, the stress of the installation of a PCIS can be the proverbial straw that breaks the camel's back. A situation in which representatives of a medical staff appear on local television to describe their boycott of the hospital and its information system as "dangerous to patient care" is just one example of how destructive this special case can be. Suffice it to say that the magnitude of effort and dedication a collaborative PCIS implementation represents demands that good lines of communication between the administration and the medical staff either exist or can be forged.

The flip side of this problem is that the stress associated with a PCIS implementation provides an excellent litmus test for the health of the medical staff–hospital relationship. The worst course of action is to ignore the history of the relationship and assume that the changes brought about by a PCIS will naturally be accepted in a hostile climate. The most effective course of action is to make use of the organizational structure suggested by this book, that is, the selection of a physician champion and a physician task force, as well as to take the time necessary to select, design, and implement a PCIS that reforges the links between the medical staff and the health care organization.

The Vocal Minority

On occasion, the minority opinion of the medical staff belongs to individuals whose stature, organizational position, or political prominence makes it difficult not to deal directly with their special agendas lest the entire PCIS project be abandoned. As discussed earlier in this chapter, the most difficult positions taken by physicians are those of computerphobia or computermania, which divert the focus of the PCIS away from the enhancement of patient care.

Although computerphobes and computermaniacs must be responded to with special attention, the amount of time, effort, and dollars poured into their special concerns must be carefully evaluated. The physician champion clearly must not come from either orientation. Instead, he or she should seek to create enough peer pressure to allow the majority staff opinion of "let's see and evaluate" come to the surface. For example, the champion could encourage the clinically influential members of the physician task force to discuss issues outside formal meeting times with members of the vocal minority. Often this form of peer pressure effectively cancels out the influence of naysayers when the soapbox has been removed.

Summary

This chapter has reviewed some of the more common maladaptive reactions to a PCIS from not only physicians but also information systems specialists and the administration of the health care organization. Among the solutions are effective communication, including well-planned educational activities and written communications; the judicious use of peer pressure; the promotion of a "service" attitude among the information management team; and, whenever appropriate, one-on-one interaction between physicians and persons who are well acquainted with the benefits of the system, whether they be information systems specialists, nurses, or other physicians.

Two of the most important elements of a successful PCIS project are, of course, the design and implementation of the PCIS itself. These topics, and an approach to the selection of a suitable information system, are discussed in chapter 4.

Information System Selection, Design, and Implementation

This chapter discusses the special issues that physician utilization of an information system raises in terms of selection, design, and implementation.

Information System Selection

The selection of an information system is a three-part process that involves:

1. Choosing a PCIS selection committee that includes physician members.
2. Learning about PCISs through vendor demonstrations and site visits. This enables the committee to define physician requirements by asking the right questions.
3. Making the closest possible match between the institution's requirements and systems currently available from PCIS vendors.

Choosing the PCIS Selection Committee

Early physician involvement in PCIS selection is extremely important. Early physician involvement sends the message of administration–physician collaboration for the life of the project. To give structure to that collaboration, an information system selection committee must be formed at this early time.

The quality of representation on this committee will have a great effect on how the issues of system functionality and operation are discussed as the project moves forward. Besides the physician champion, the selection committee should include a representative or representatives from the medical staff leadership. The committee also should include the CIO of the health care organization (or director of information systems or data processing), the CFO, the chief nursing officer (CNO), and other strategic administrative leaders. As discussed in chapter 2, it is important that the representative(s) of the medical staff leadership be chosen from the ranks of clinically *influential* physicians, whether they are department chairs or not.

From the outset of the project, the selection committee's composition and deliberations should be communicated widely to set the tone that the medical staff's ownership and involvement have been sought from the beginning. Some health care leaders have rejected this approach for fear of creating too large a committee or somehow losing control of the process. Obviously, certain negotiations must be kept confidential until contracts have been developed. However, the communication of ongoing, major issues of concern to the medical staff can act as a powerful validation of the direction being taken by this important body.

Learning about PCISs

Educating the PCIS selection committee is the first important task facing this group. The education process includes vendor demonstrations and site visits. The CIO or data processing director can perform an important role here as education facilitator, enlightening all members of the selection committee regarding current system capabilities and the potential for future capabilities. From the perspective of the selection of a PCIS designed for direct physician use, there are special considerations for each of these education processes.

Vendor Demonstrations

The selection of which vendors to invite to the hospital to give a demonstration is usually the responsibility of the CIO or the information systems director. The list of vendors is usually drawn up on the basis of what kind of system is being sought (clinical, financial, or other) and the size of the health care organization or system to be served. The ability of vendors to successfully respond to the committee's preliminary questions should help the committee determine whether the vendor list requires expansion. The five major questions the committee should ask are as follows:

1. *Is the vendor's system designed for direct use by physicians?* The vendor's answer to this question should contain a number of elements:
   - Clinical input used to design its system
   - Degree of user customization possible to meet special clinical needs
   - Attention to how clinicians would actually use the system for patient care (for example, method of information entry and retrieval, use during patient rounds, speed of system operation)
   - Amount of clinical information held in the system that is necessary for patient care (see the discussion of the electronic patient record in question #5)
   - Degree to which the system supports inpatient and outpatient activities
   - Degree to which on-line information is organized in a clinically logical manner (for example, problem oriented, diagnosis related)

- Degree to which the system assists the physician in performing daily activities (for example, work lists, automatic drug dosage calculations, information on drug interactions, clinical reminders)
- Degree to which the system allows clinicians to review their own clinical performance by patient, diagnosis-related group (DRG), and therapy (including capability for clinical research)
- Method by which the system provides for security safeguards in support of the patient's rights and the confidentiality of the physician–patient relationship

2. *Is the system actually being used by physicians for day-to-day patient care? If so, where? Can the selection committee see this application for themselves?* Watch for signs of stress in the vendor after asking these questions. In contradistinction to the claims and hyperbole that accompany any sales effort, the answer to the final question must be either yes or no. The proof of the validity of any of the claims made in a vendor demonstration or in response to the first question is whether the theory behind a particular PCIS has been applied in practice. The response here should satisfy the primary considerations for deciding whether to make any site visits in the near future.

3. *Has the system been proven to meet clinical demands?* The true computer demands of a 24-hour-a-day, 365-day-a-year fault-intolerant service such as patient care are extreme. Some older information systems are only patched-together financial computing systems that, although they may have the strict requirements for accuracy, do not have the speed of operation and flexibility demanded from a PCIS. These requirements of speed and flexibility warrant further consideration.

The PCIS is expected to be a communication tool interconnecting, facilitating, and accelerating the delivery of high-quality patient care. A PCIS that gets in the way of physician ordering and results retrieval because of either poor, nonintuitive design or slow response time will not be accepted by clinicians and will not yield the expected benefits of enhancing patient care delivery. Therefore, a successful PCIS must not only be easy to use but must also enhance the *speed* with which physicians can go about their daily work.

Flexibility speaks to the ability of the PCIS to present different capabilities to different users and to be easily modified to do so. The antithesis of this is the rigidly structured information system that requires weeks of work to achieve even the most elementary changes, such as those in the formatting of screen information. As noted in the next section, two questions that a site visit should answer are: (1) How long does it take for changes to be made to the PCIS? and (2) How has the system affected the daily rounds of physicians? A site visit should answer questions about system flexibility and speed.

4. *How does the vendor incorporate the experiences that clinicians have had with the system at other institutions into the product the vendor*

is planning to offer? The physician task force can be far more effective and productive when the PCIS selection committee presents it with choices instead of asking it to "reinvent the wheel" when it comes to configuring and customizing an information system. Furthermore, a company that continues to sell a system for its possibilities rather than its delivered capabilities appears to be resting on past laurels and to have little interest in growth, development, and innovation. From the vendor's standpoint, delivering prepackaged, so-called turnkey systems also is undesirable and appears to be trying to shoehorn all its users into operating alike. The balance struck between these two extremes is often quite revealing in terms of how vendors actually view their products and their clients.

5. *What is the scope and design of this vendor's version of the electronic patient record?* The vendor's response to this question can illumine several important issues:

   • Is this product touted as doing all things for all people or as an open, "architectured" system with interconnections to other systems now and in the future? In the information industry, most players have realized that monolithic systems cannot be all things to all people. The future will belong to those vendors who recognize the vital considerations of building interfaces and offering support for distributed information processing. For example, the selection committee should find out whether clinical information transfer standards (such as HL7) are supported by the PCIS vendor. If not, the ability to connect to future information tools may be limited.

   • Has the vendor seriously considered its product's use as an active patient care record? If the vendor has not given sufficient thought to developing a patient care record, it may be difficult to configure the product to operate as an electronic patient record in a particular institution. In addition, ask the vendor whether the product is expected to operate as an abstract of the written medical record or replace it entirely.

   • Does the patient care record have continuity for both inpatient and outpatient settings? For the next several years, the strategic initiatives of U.S. hospitals and health care enterprises will include networking with physicians' offices and other outpatient services. To be clinically useful, information tools must support the collection and communication of the entire patient record, including inpatient and outpatient activities.

Satisfactory answers to these and the other major questions in this section may lead the PCIS selection committee to request a vendor to demonstrate its product. The design, development, and execution of vendor demonstrations is an art in itself. Considering the cost of the products being sold, it is surprising that demonstrations are not more professional and polished and designed for the needs of the audience. In fairness to the vendors, however, it is unusual for a selection committee to provide detailed information on what members would like to see in a system demonstration, preferring instead to "see what they've got." As a result, most demonstrations dazzle but fail to inform. Although exhaustive requests for proposals (RFPs) are unnecessary before inviting vendor demonstrations, far more information can be exchanged if the PCIS selection committee develops a list of basic requirements. Those requirements can be communicated as part of a request for information, or RFI.

The RFI allows health care institutions to identify for vendors their vital statistics, current information systems capabilities, and wants and needs for the proposed information system. Vendors respond to an RFI by stating company history, product lines, client lists, references, features and functions, service capabilities, and approximate prices. The streamlined RFI can be a useful tool in determining which vendors should be given serious consideration. Other information on vendors can be gathered at professional meetings and vendor exhibitions, in journals, and through normal collegial networking.

An interesting trend in vendor demonstrations is the *current user demo.* Such demonstrations are conducted by current system users from other institutions and sometimes can provide important insights into what is actually achievable by using the product. For the purpose of this discussion, a demonstration by a physician user from another hospital can be ideal for communicating to the selection committee how real clinicians can make effective use of a particular PCIS product. Because the demonstrator will likely be talking in language familiar to physicians, the "noncomputerese" style of communication can therefore be the best way to educate committee members regarding the use of a particular system.

The combination of holding a demonstration by an articulate, informed current user and asking the right questions of the vendor can make the best use of the selection committee's time. Not only will the committee be able to plan effective site visits, but it will also find the selection process to be significantly easier.

Site Visits

Site visits by the PCIS selection committee (or a subset of it) are common practice prior to the selection of a PCIS. In the current cost-containment climate, junkets of large groups to hospital sites are undesirable and can rapidly eat up budgets. However, carefully chosen and organized site visits can be invaluable in making believers out of the committee members and can begin the process of change at a health care organization. If the vendor sites can be selected in response to the second major question posed above

(Is the system actually being used by physicians for patient care?), important insights may be obtained regarding the staff's ability to process change and the real advantages of a particular PCIS at the institution.

Several things to look for at a site visit are:

1. Who is actually using the PCIS?
2. Are alternate methods of communication (telephones, other computer systems, and so forth) being used more or less often than the PCIS being demonstrated?
3. What does a physician user who was not selected by the vendor to take part in the site visit think of the PCIS? How does the system really work for him or her?
4. Can a medical chart generated by the PCIS actually be used for day-to-day patient care?
5. How interested are physician users in having this PCIS in their offices?

The site visit needs of the physician champion are somewhat different from those of the selection committee as a whole. The physician champion should consider the following questions when evaluating sites:

1. Is this institution similar to your own in size, demographics, structure of the medical staff (open/closed), and training program?
2. To what extent do physicians really use the information system at this institution? How do the physicians say the system has affected their daily rounds?
3. What departments have most successfully implemented the PCIS at this site?
4. Do the departments that have been unsuccessful provide an important object lesson that needs to be communicated to the selection committee (that is, the necessity for early involvement of staff, the ability to customize the information tools to fit the users, the importance of good management of change in the department, and so on)?
5. According to the PCIS director at the site, how long does it take to make changes to the information system?
6. Is the PCIS director willing to customize the tour to meet your needs, including arranging specific interviews with physician users?

Making the Closest Possible Match

The process of matching a particular institution's information needs with information systems available on the market is an inexact science and is beyond the scope of this discussion. Nevertheless, informed physicians need to remain active in this process as the committee moves toward a final selection. Clinical and administrative considerations should intermingle in the selection committee's deliberations to achieve the best possible choice for an institution's specific future information needs.

It is at this juncture that some physicians decide that their needs will remain unmet by any available vendor's information system. The temptation is to consider designing a system from scratch. Unfortunately, in today's environment the trend toward do-it-yourself information systems appears to be over, given the current constraints on resources and costs. In certain settings, such as university hospitals, local resources may indeed be available that ultimately better serve the institution's needs. But today, even such settings are reconsidering the do-it-yourself approach in favor of flexible, commercially available PCISs, because of both economic and time constraints. Thus, it is wise to think more than twice before succumbing to the allure of the "we-can-do-it-better-here" syndrome!

As mentioned earlier, one tool that has been used in making a vendor selection is the RFP. The RFP has traditionally asked vendors to provide information on system capabilities, costs, installation, support, and other essential data on why a particular system may best meet the needs of an institution. Written vendor responses, which can take several weeks to prepare, enable the selection committee to compare various systems and reach a decision to buy.

A formal RFP process may still be useful to some institutions, but most information systems executives agree that the detailed responses utilized in the past (and even required by some institutions) yielded few practical benefits. Today, health care executives and vendor representatives are more knowledgeable, sophisticated, and efficient, and contract negotiations can begin and conclude in a shorter period of time for the betterment of all parties.

System Design

Following the choice of a vendor by the PCIS selection committee, the physician task force and the PCIS management group within the information systems department become involved in the design of an efficient PCIS. For the purposes of this discussion, *PCIS design* refers to the process of modifying a vendor's system to meet the form and functional requirements of a particular institution.

An example of a *form requirement* is a hospital's formulary. No two hospital formularies are exactly alike, and if your PCIS is to allow pharmacy ordering on-line, it must contain all the medications in your formulary.

An example of a *functional requirement* is the handling of an order for an arterial blood gas measurement. In some hospitals, the respiratory therapist obtains the arterial blood gas sample, but the chemistry laboratory actually runs the test on it. The functional requirement for a PCIS in this situation would be to transmit a request for the blood draw to the respiratory therapy department and send a separate notice to run the test on the specimen to the lab, preferably after the therapist has obtained the blood. Appropriate status messages would be created on-line, first, to let the physician and the nurse know that the blood had been collected and the specimen was being tested by the lab, and, second, to report the results.

System design to meet the form and functional requirements of the health care organization is a three-part process:

1. Data collection
2. System modification
3. Functional and integrated system testing

Data collection in this context refers to the gathering of information from the various physician groups on what design will best meet their needs.

System modification is the more technical process of coding the information system to meet the requirements defined in the data collection process.

Functional testing is the process whereby each individual element of the information system is tested for efficacy of performance. For example, if your hospital's information system is divided into pharmacy, laboratory, nursing, physician, and other modules, each module is tested on an individual basis.

Integrated testing is the testing of all the modules together as well as the interfaces to other information systems with which the PCIS must communicate (for example, the patient accounting system, the executive information system, and so on).

Data Collection

Data collection is the process of identifying, analyzing, and documenting the form and functional requirements of each and every patient care delivery division and department in an institution. The details of this substantial task are beyond the scope of this book. However, the role the physician task force plays in the data collection process is crucial to the success of a PCIS installation that anticipates direct physician use.

The physician task force participates in the data collection process in two ways: by providing clinical oversight, and by having members serve as primary data collectors.

The majority of the task force's data collection work is clinical oversight. *Clinical oversight* consists of reviewing the form and functional specifications identified by the various departments and resolving the differences between how departments want to receive orders and report results and how clinicians need to enter and process this information.

For example, the radiology department may wish to call a standard chest X ray a frontal chest X ray, whereas most clinicians may call the same film a PA (posterior–anterior) chest X ray. Because clinician familiarity with radiology ordering is the paramount concern, the data collection form would be modified by the physician task force to reflect the clinicians' favored terminology. This same logic would apply to pharmacy and nursing specifications for the PCIS, so that the physicians would find the information system easy to use.

Frequently, in the process of data collection the physician task force will identify issues regarding the use of the PCIS that will significantly affect clinical practice. Physicians in one particular nursing unit may have placed orders using special phrases known only to certain nurses (for example, "magic mouthwash" or "my postop package"). These terms are imprecise at best, and when directly transmitted via a PCIS to the pharmacy or laboratory, they are meaningless. It is important that the physician task force identify these issues and negotiate changes in clinical practice early in the design process.

The physician task force acts as a primary data collector regarding physician practice-specific issues. For example, standard practice protocols specific to procedures (such as surgical subspecialties) or practices (such as hematology/oncology chemotherapy protocols) must be defined and included in the design of a PCIS in order to support clinical practice in these areas. Physician clinical experts in these areas can play an early and significant role in the development of the PCIS simply by writing out these protocols. Our experience in this aspect of physician involvement suggests that most clinicians are willing to cooperate and are honored that their clinical guidelines are being incorporated into the PCIS.

System Modification

System modification, or the technical process of information system coding to meet the requirements defined in the data collection process, is rarely the responsibility of either the physician champion or the physician task force. Nevertheless, excellent and consistent communication between the technical information systems experts and the physician task force is important to avoid excessive iterations of system coding. It may be helpful, therefore, to acquaint the physician champion with an overview of the issues involved in technical system modification. In this manner, the physician champion can act as a more effective translator of clinical issues into the technical experts' language, thereby benefiting both groups.

Functional and Integrated System Testing

Functional and integrated system testing provides the first medical-staffwide opportunity for physician involvement. System testing of both the individual departmental components (functional testing) and the system as a whole (integrated testing) is most often coordinated by the information systems department.

Details of this process are beyond the scope of this book. However, the process of testing requires a number of participants. Therefore, it may be advisable to include physicians in the testing process who have not yet had the opportunity to view the system, thereby offering them a kind of sneak preview.

Although these "testing" physicians will need more orientation in order to act effectively in the test role, the orientation will serve to disseminate an awareness of PCIS capabilities among the medical staff. In addition, the orientation will have begun a process of enhancing physician sensitivity to the complexity of the PCIS and its interconnections with other computer systems (that is, its interfaces). This "sensitivity training" can yield important dividends later in PCIS implementation, because as requests for system changes arise, physicians who have an understanding of the system will better appreciate the time and effort it takes to make those changes.

System Implementation

The implementation of a PCIS is the process of introducing the system throughout an enterprise, including inpatient, outpatient, and physician office locations. Three aspects of implementation, particularly important from the physician's point of view, are discussed in the remainder of this chapter:

1. The method of implementation
2. The education of physicians
3. Physician support during PCIS implementation

The Method of Implementation

The method of implementing a PCIS can have an important effect on physician acceptance and use of the system. The most important rule of thumb is to customize the implementation approach for your medical staff and hospital setting. Although numerous variations exist, there are two main styles of implementation: the partial, or "wave," method; and the big bang method. Each method has distinct advantages and disadvantages from the perspectives of both the physician and the institution.

The Partial, or "Wave," Method

The partial, or "wave," method of implementation is defined as the introduction of the PCIS in sections. For example, a wave implementation of a PCIS could involve introducing the system into one department at a time (one wave of implementation at a time), with each and every area of the organization on-line with that one department at the same time. Thus the laboratory portion of the PCIS could be introduced organizationwide, followed by the radiology portion, the pharmacy portion, and so on.

The primary advantages of this method of implementation are: (1) a slower change in the day-to-day activities of physicians and nurses (that is, one part of PCIS to deal with at a time); and (2) an easier implementation for departments, because either they are fully "up" on the PCIS or they are not (that is, there are fewer duplicate systems for the ancillaries).

There are two disadvantages of this method. First, the implementation process is more difficult for physicians and nurses because duplicate systems (for example, paper orders for some departments and computerized orders for others) are retained longer on nursing units. Second, this type of implementation involves an increased risk of rejection by physicians and nurses. That is, the more difficult portions of the PCIS and the easier-to-adjust-to portions of the PCIS are not perceived as a whole.

This second disadvantage requires further explanation. Regardless of what type of PCIS has been selected and how expertly its functioning has been modified to meet the needs of the institution and its medical staff, the introduction of the PCIS will still cause a profound change in the day-to-day operations of clinicians and staff. As was discussed in earlier chapters, a full order-entry and results-reporting PCIS contains some features that, by the nature of the activity involved, will be easier to use than others. (For example, laboratory orders will be easier to use than pharmacy order entry and charting.) If the wave method of implementation is chosen, staff and clinicians may reject the introduction of the more difficult features of the system and wish to use only the easier ones. They will not have had the opportunity to see and accept the PCIS as a whole automation-induced change to their day-to-day activities, and they will not appreciate the importance of accepting initial delays in implementing one portion of the PCIS.

For example, physicians may object to direct order entry for one implemented department's portion of the PCIS because they continually need to remember which ones can still be written and which ones must be entered via the computer. This additional and unnatural burden on the communication duties of clinicians (that is, ordering) may significantly and negatively affect physician acceptance of the PCIS.

The Big Bang Method

The big bang method is defined as the introduction of the entire functionality of the PCIS, one nursing unit at a time. That is, when a nursing area, outpatient clinic, and so forth, comes "up" on the PCIS, each is given all the on-line departments and features at the same time.

This method of implementation has several advantages. First, there is only one large change for clinicians and it is consistent for all activities on that nursing unit. Second, physicians, nurses, and staff see and evaluate the entire PCIS at once and thus gain a better understanding of the overall benefits to their daily work of the different portions of the system. And third, ancillary departments (for example, lab, pharmacy, and so on) experience fewer changes in their operations at a time (that is, only one nursing unit moves on-line at a time).

This method also has some disadvantages. First, it requires more resources for training, user support, and technical support (that is, all sections of the PCIS must be fully completed for implementation of the first nursing unit). Second, it duplicates systems (paper and computer) in ancillary departments for a longer period of time while the implementation proceeds throughout the rest of the health care organization. And third, if staff and management are not up to the challenge, the single large change in day-to-day operations may be overwhelming.

Choosing a Method of Implementation

Which method of PCIS implementation should you choose? After balancing the relative strengths and weaknesses of your institution and medical staff against the relative advantages and disadvantages of each method, you should be able to identify which method best meets your needs.

If your medical staff and institution are up to it, we recommend the big bang method because the ability of physicians to absorb the change to daily activities that the PCIS brings is directly proportional to their understanding of the total benefits they receive from the change. Until a PCIS arrives on the market that accepts and understands naturally connected speech from all users, the narrow process of writing orders will always be faster with pen and paper than with keyboard, light pen, or mouse for most physicians. Therefore, it is preferable that the whole of the PCIS be available from the start so that physicians can see the benefits of the other time-savers and effort-savers the system can provide.

Choosing the First Nursing Unit to Implement the PCIS

Another implementation issue is how to select the first nursing area to come on-line with your PCIS. The primary consideration here is which nursing area and physician group are best able to absorb the change of PCIS introduction. The importance of selecting the first unit well is obvious, because nothing can plague an implementation more than an initial failure. Consider the following questions and issues when making your decision:

1. Which nursing area has best dealt with previous operational changes (for example, changes in hospital procedures, forms, and so on)?

2. Which nursing area has the best reputation for close collaboration between physicians and nurses?
3. Which nursing area has the most capable nursing supervisor?
4. Which nursing area has a nursing staff that has been working well together for the longest time?
5. Which nursing area has the most stable clinical operation (that is, fewer transfers, similar types of patients, and a stable group of physicians using that area)?

Although the fifth consideration is not as important as the other four, stability will nevertheless make it more likely that the area will accept the PCIS with minimal difficulty.

The Education of Physicians

Physician education is a vital part of a PCIS implementation plan, but it is balanced on the razor's edge of two competing forces: (1) the amount of information you want to impart to the physician; and (2) the amount of time the average physician has to spend in PCIS training. For the purposes of our discussion, this issue can be separated into two parts: (1) methods of physician training on a PCIS; and (2) physician training guidelines.

Methods of Physician Training

Although numerous possible methods exist for physician PCIS training, several are especially worthy of further consideration:

- Group training
- One-on-one instruction
- Independent instruction

After a brief description of each method, some of the advantages and disadvantages of each are listed.

Group Training

Group training refers to physician training in a classroom setting involving four or more physicians per instructor. The group of physicians is usually provided with written instructional materials and individual access to a computer terminal when practical demonstration and drilling are necessary.

The advantages of group training are:

- It allows physicians to learn in the company of their peers (collaboration), exchanging issues, techniques, and problem solving on the spot (for example, how to use the system in their group's practice style).

- It ensures the efficient use of time by the training personnel.
- It provides a consistent message to several physicians at one time.
- It is probably the most successful technique for instructing physicians-in-training, that is, residents and medical students.

The disadvantages of group training are:

- Not all physicians in a group will learn the techniques at the same rate. (It could be intimidating for a physician to admit this in the company of his or her professional colleagues.)
- It is difficult to call a consistent group of physicians together for training, which dilutes the collaborative advantage.
- This method ignores special practice needs.
- It is difficult to accommodate the time constraints of busy practitioners.

One-on-One Instruction

One-on-one instruction is a method whereby one instructor is assigned to one physician. This represents the ultimate in personalized instruction. It usually includes training materials customized for the individual physician and a personalized certification examination (described later in this chapter). The advantages of one-on-one instruction are:

- It offers the best flexibility for the timing and location of training sessions for the physician who does not desire independent instruction (see next section). One-on-one instruction is ideal for clinically influential physicians who must be certified prior to system activation.
- It builds a strong understanding/support relationship between the physician and the instructor.
- A personalized certification examination ensures that the physician will be able to perform on-line all the necessary activities that he or she will need to carry out daily clinical duties.

The disadvantages are:

- This method involves the least efficient use of training personnel time (that is, fewer physicians are trained per unit of instructor time).
- Because of inevitable resource limitations, this method can be provided to only a select few physicians.

Independent Instruction

Independent instruction, or self-paced learning, involves the use of training materials by the individual physician, who is free to determine the time and place of his or her training, as well as the duration. A more recent development in this mode of instruction is computer-assisted instruction, or CAI, which allows the physician to use a computer program to walk through the on-line lessons in the use of a PCIS at his or her own pace. The computer can show the actual screens from the real PCIS in a safe environment at the time and place most convenient for the physician—even at home! The carefully constructed CAI system will also be customized for the particular physician, presenting only the necessary information for proficiency on the PCIS for that physician's practice. The certification examination can be performed within the CAI program and returned to the PCIS instructor for verification and password assignment.

The advantages of independent instruction are:

- It provides the ultimate in flexibility of time, location, and pace of the training experience, because all are controlled by the individual.
- It ensures maximal efficiency of instructor time, because the individual PCIS instructor can assist many physicians at the same time with CAI.
- Its individualization of instructional features is equal to the one-on-one method.

The disadvantages are:

- Depending on the power of the CAI program, this method is probably not as interactive as a human can be in one-on-one instruction.
- If CAI instruction is not properly managed by the PCIS instructor, the time to achieve certification can be prolonged.
- Initial development time for a superior CAI program is greater than for development of written materials alone.

Physician Training Guidelines

Three guidelines for physician training must be kept in mind to ensure optimum results from the training process. These guidelines were alluded to in the previous discussion but warrant further explanation:

1. A PCIS certification examination should be developed and administered.
2. Physicians should be supported during the training process.
3. The training experience should be customized to the needs of the individual physician.

To ensure the effectiveness and safety of physicians on-line, the first guideline is that a certification examination should be developed and administered to each physician prior to assigning an on-line PCIS password, regardless of which method of training is chosen. The certification examination may be written or, in the case of CAI, computerized. The examination should be customized for the elements of the PCIS that a particular physician is most likely to use. Obviously, all information should be kept confidential by the PCIS instructor, and retesting should always be allowed after some remedial instruction.

Second, physician-training support is necessary regardless of the method of training chosen. Because of the limitations of a busy clinician's schedule, further training support should be available in some manner after normal business hours (for example, by appointment). The key words here are *flexibility* and *service*. A section of the information systems staff devoted to PCIS physician instruction needs to exhibit both of these qualities, thereby delivering that all-important good first impression that the PCIS project always needs.

The final guideline addresses the customization of the training experience. To the extent that special care is taken not to educate a physician to perform a clinical task that he or she will never need to perform, that physician will feel that the instruction and the PCIS are relevant to his or her practice. For example, if a physician who has not ordered intravenous hyperalimentation solution since medical school is now presented with his or her first practical example of using the PCIS by writing "hyperal" orders, that physician will naturally feel the training experience to be a waste of time. The appropriate functions and activities that should be taught can be arrived at through negotiation with the individual physician or, as in the case of CAI, through allowing menu selection of the relevant portions of the PCIS for instruction.

Physician Support during PCIS Implementation

Physician support both during and after PCIS implementation is a key element of successful achievement of direct physician use of both the order-entry and results-reporting capabilities of a PCIS system. The process of physician support is complex and involves the efforts of a dedicated team. The remainder of this chapter discusses the membership and responsibilities of the physician support team and the problem-solving process.

The Physician Support Team

PCIS physician user support is a collaborative process involving the physician champion, members of the PCIS physician task force, nursing special users who have been educated to know how the new PCIS works, ancillary department special users, and information systems support personnel.

The physician champion can act as a focal point or "one-stop service" for physician support by being available on implemented nursing units by page, and even on-line via electronic mail. This aspect of the physician champion's job is a natural extension of the authority and responsibility that the hospital administration and medical staff imbued him or her with at the beginning of the project. To the extent that access to support is made easy, quick, and efficient, physicians will use the vehicles for the support available to them. Thus the physician champion must continue to act as the conduit for PCIS problems and issues that require resolution.

The physician champion may also coordinate user support by calling together and conducting pre-implementation user support meetings. These meetings allow all users (including physicians, nurses, secretaries, and others) on each soon-to-be-activated nursing unit to express concerns and issues, as well as to plan how they will support one another through the changes brought about by PCIS implementation.

The members of the PCIS physician task force play another important role in user support. They are the special physician users who have greater knowledge of the system than other physicians who are still completing their certification training. Task force members also may act as ambassadors for the system, explaining how the PCIS works and how other physicians can best adjust their daily clinical rounds and activities to make optimal use of the system.

Special nurse users are a front line of support for residents and attending physicians in the nursing areas. These nurses have several special advantages as PCIS physician supporters:

- They have a working knowledge of both physician practice patterns and PCIS operation.
- They are personally familiar with the physicians practicing in their nursing unit.
- They are physically available on the nursing unit when a physician's questions first arise (thus, they can minimize frustration when problems occur).
- They can act as coordinators of support services for physicians from ancillary departments (for example, pharmacy, laboratory, and so on) and from the information systems department.

In fact, an excellent structural model of physician user support is to have ancillary department and information systems support personnel work through the special nurse user. In this way, the special nurse user filters the clinically and operationally important information to be communicated back to the physician, a role that many nurses already fulfill in the nonautomated nursing unit.

Ancillary department special users are the topic experts in their division for the PCIS. For example, the pharmacy special user will most likely be a pharmacist who knows exactly how the PCIS works in his or her area and is able to solve the problems other users may be having with that portion of the PCIS. As previously discussed, this individual works best through the nursing special user in supporting physician use of the PCIS.

Information systems support personnel are experts in the technical support of PCIS operation and have ultimate responsibility for the proper operation of the system's hardware (such as printers and terminals). Physicians and other users must have ready access to this support group in the event of apparent equipment failure. The urgency of this direct contact is engendered by the fact that the PCIS is a *clinical* information system. Patient care is reliant on the communications that this system facilitates; hence time is always a critical factor.

The Problem-Solving Process

Even in a small health care organization, the process of identifying, tracking, and processing PCIS problems is a large task. Although a comprehensive discussion of PCIS problem processing is beyond the scope of this book, several guidelines are particularly relevant to physicians and their use of the PCIS: (1) ensure "front-end" access; (2) maintain a problem-tracking mechanism; and (3) ensure that solutions to problems are broadly communicated to users.

Front-end access for problem solving means that physicians must have a simple way to access the problem-solving process. The physician champion may be this access point; however, all staff involved in the support process must view user (customer) service as the paramount consideration in all user interactions. The most effective means of alienating physicians (or any other group) from the PCIS is to present the frustrated user with a labyrinthine bureaucracy each and every time a problem is posed.

Problem-tracking mechanism refers to the means for selecting and maintaining a common-access roster of problems for all support personnel throughout the life of the information system. This may take the form of a written problem roster or a complex, networked database. What is most important is that the tracking method avoid reinventing solutions each time the same problem is presented, thereby avoiding a situation in which numerous personnel are solving the same problem at the same time. Further, a problem-tracking mechanism should provide a means for sending a progress report to the requesting user (physician or other staff member) at regular intervals to avoid the impression that all requests are swallowed into a black hole.

Problem/solution communication should be well integrated into the ongoing communications from the PCIS project staff to the medical staff. All too often, the PCIS project staff misses a prime opportunity to enhance public (user) relations by not broadly communicating that, thanks to the cooperation of the physician users and the PCIS support team, a difficult issue has been resolved and the patient care operation is all the better for it.

Summary

This chapter has reviewed the special considerations for selecting, designing, and implementing a PCIS that is intended for direct use by physicians. Of course, any physician task force and PCIS selection committee will have many additional concerns for and requirements of a PCIS and the various system vendors. However, the procedures and questions posed by this chapter should help clarify from the very beginning of your deliberations the true clinical utility of the systems being considered.

Clearly, one of the most important information connections for a PCIS is between the hospital and the physician's office. This connection, a potentially vital tool for physician practice, is the topic of chapter 5.

Chapter Five

Physician Office Links: The Real Network

There is growing interest among U.S. hospitals in delivering PCISs directly into physicians' offices. Because of the significant implications of this trend for maximizing the patient care benefits of a PCIS and achieving the strategic initiatives that prompted the purchase of the PCIS to begin with, this topic deserves special comment.

For the purpose of this discussion, *PCIS-networked physician offices* refers to the connection between a hospital-based PCIS and area physicians' offices. These links provide two-way communication between hospital and office with or without direct communication links between physician offices. In addition to ordering, results-reporting, and patient-scheduling capabilities, these systems also contain full electronic mail functionality.

Advantages to the Hospital

To understand the current interest in linking physicians' offices to a PCIS, the motivations of the two primary participants, the hospital administration and the physicians, need to be evaluated. From the hospital administration's standpoint, physician office links with a PCIS have several major advantages: (1) they help accomplish strategic initiatives; (2) they improve physician bonding; (3) they enhance physician use of the PCIS; (4) they improve the PCIS database; and (5) they enhance communication between hospitals and physicians.

Accomplishment of Strategic Initiatives

The PCIS provides an instrument for the accomplishment of many strategic initiatives. Within the context of this discussion, key among these initiatives is physician networking. In the current economic and regulatory climate in U.S. health care, many hospitals are "circling the wagons," that is, creating hospital systems and forging other interinstitutional relationships. The stimulus for this health care trend is the belief that consolidation during difficult economic times enhances the prospects for survival of all hospitals, both large and small.

One of the enticements for smaller institutions to consolidate is the gain in equipment and technology that would otherwise not be available to them. A PCIS is one obvious example. A well-designed and well-executed PCIS can be the principal attraction for an entire medical staff to join a health system. For an individual physician, a networked PCIS installed in his or her office can serve as an enticement to refer to a tertiary care hospital because of the ease of communication to and from the electronically linked sites. Therefore, a PCIS may be offered by a hospital administration as an enticement to other institutions to collaborate and even consolidate on the basis of extended physician office networking.

Improvement in Physician Bonding

Physician bonding refers to the process whereby a hospital administration attracts and develops a loyal medical staff. In the current era of interhospital competition, this process can be crucial to a hospital's continued success, and even survival. The PCIS can enhance physician bonding to an institution via several mechanisms:

- Improved quality of practice
- Value-added aspects of practicing and using the PCIS-based institution
- Enhanced practice efficiency

Improved quality of practice refers to the advantages to clinical practice arising from the use of a PCIS (see chapter 1) in terms of quality enhancements such as automatic drug interaction alerts, improved electronic medical record legibility, and effective order communication. A properly designed and executed PCIS simply makes it easier to practice good medicine.

Value-added aspects of the PCIS refers to the additional information that a PCIS provides to physicians that would otherwise be either unavailable or difficult to find. This information includes clinical, financial, and demographic data.

In terms of clinical data, a PCIS would give physicians immediate access to clinical data from any interaction that a patient had had within the health care system. This would include lab tests, X rays, clinical summaries (for example, discharge summaries, operative reports), and even progress notes. Without a PCIS clinicians would see only a portion of this information at a time.

In terms of financial and demographic data, a PCIS would normally contain the pertinent billing and insurance information associated with each encounter. If the PCIS is distributed to physicians' offices, the physicians may share access to this information, which would greatly decrease registration and billing processing time. Demographic information would be collected once and used for all of the various documentation and billing forms that have become part of U.S. health care. This access provides significant benefits for the physician, his or her staff, and the patient in terms of the time and effort normally associated with gathering such information.

Enhanced practice efficiency refers to the advantages the PCIS offers physicians in terms of saving time and facilitating procedures and communication in the office. These include: patient appointment scheduling, with a window to all the available services the medical center offers; remote-access inpatient and outpatient information, enabling the busy clinician to keep track of patient status while in the office; and electronic mail, which enables the physician to efficiently make important contacts with other physicians and administration and avoid the frustration of playing telephone tag.

Enhanced Physician Use of Information Systems

Considering the total investment a health care organization makes in a PCIS, it is essential to maximize effective system use by physicians to achieve the expected benefits (see chapter 2). A physician office link to a PCIS provides strong incentives for increased physician utilization of the entire information system at several levels. First, the physician's office staff usually strongly advocates obtaining the value-added information available on a PCIS in the office. Second, the major benefit of remote information access and ordering is realized only when an office system is installed, making it more important for the physician to learn and use the PCIS. Third, a PCIS integrated with the physician's office database provides important communication and patient care information to the clinician when he or she needs it during rounds, in the emergency room, and so forth.

Improvement of the PCIS Database

Improvement of the PCIS database refers to the enhanced value of the database when it is more inclusive of all inpatient and outpatient activities. Security and access issues notwithstanding, a truly complete record of all patient visits and patient care—including inpatient and outpatient care, emergency services, and physician office care—significantly enhances the value of the electronic patient record for all purposes. In fact, without full patient record continuity, the patient care, clinical research, quality assurance, and utilization review advantages of the system are diminished.

Enhanced Communication

Communication between hospital administration and physician offices is vital to the successful operation of any medical institution. Unfortunately, the traditional methods of memos and mail make this information link tenuous at best. The PCIS-delivered electronic mail functionality can have a profound effect on the consistency and quality of the information exchange between the organization and the physician's office. Changes in organization policy, formulary, and operations can be rapidly disseminated throughout the physician community, thus avoiding the often costly and time-consuming process of chasing down busy clinicians via telephone. The timely nature of this form of mail also removes many perceived barriers to access between clinicians and administration.

Advantages to the Physicians

From the physician's perspective, physician office links to the PCIS provide four major advantages: (1) they improve practice efficiency; (2) they improve practice quality; (3) they provide a link to the physician's office records when he or she is working at the hospital; and (4) they provide improved billing information and resources. Improved efficiency and quality of practice were discussed in the previous section; the latter two advantages are discussed in this section.

Hospital Link to Physician Office Records

Keeping track of a patient's medications, procedures, consultations, and outpatient visits continues to constitute the majority of the data collection work of the physician. The increased mobility of today's society and the increased numbers of tests and procedures available add to the difficulty of this task. Despite the difficulty involved in the process, however, patients have every right to expect their physicians to have all this information at their fingertips when new decisions need to be made. The link between the PCIS and the physician office brings this expectation closer to reality.

The hospital-to-office link provides a common repository for all inpatient and outpatient clinical information as well as the most up-to-date listing of future planned patient care. For a busy clinical practice, the advantage provided by this electronic fix for the medical paper chase is not simply a convenience; it can mean better-quality patient care, less clinician time wasted, and decreased medical liability. Remarkably, many physicians now expect that any new PCIS will provide this type of functionality.

Physician Link to Billing Information

The strain placed on physician billing operations of small practices by the growing bureaucracy of third-party billing is growing daily. Lacking the resources of the hospital's registration and financial departments, the practicing clinician can greatly benefit from sharing billing and other information with the PCIS-based institution. In a similar fashion to the enhanced clinical functionality of networked office and hospital information systems, the medical office financial link to the hospital information system can provide important advantages to both parties. Obviously, security of information on both sides is essential, with flexible ability to provide or restrict information access as needed (see chapter 6).

Considerations for Implementation

Provided the benefits of a PCIS–physician office link are found compelling to both administration and physicians, a number of important questions must be posed: For which physicians should this office link be provided? What is actually being provided? How should security be handled? How much will it cost? This section addresses the concerns expressed by those questions.

Physician Access

Important new federal regulations now specifically prohibit hospitals from providing free services to physicians on the basis of numbers of patients admitted or referred (Medicare/Medicaid/Title V/Title XX Anti-Fraud and Abuse Amendments, Social Security Act 1128B(b), 42 U.S.C. 1320a-7b). Therefore, the decision to provide links between a PCIS and physicians' offices must be provided without prejudice, and equal access to these systems must be ensured. Obviously, the scope of what is provided, and the internal hospital structure for providing it and supporting the services, must take this issue into account. In reality, it is likely that the initial group of physicians interested in having office links with a hospital PCIS will include those physicians who already frequently use that hospital's services. If these pilot sites are successful, the process of physician attraction and bonding may well extend outside this core group. Suffice it to say that the first impression of the functionality and benefits of this linkage will be communicated rapidly throughout the physician community, making planning and preparation even more important.

Functionality

A wide range of possible links between the PCIS and physicians' offices can be reviewed up to and including the ideal definition at the beginning of this chapter. These possibilities include the following stages: (1) placement of a PCIS terminal in each physician's office; (2) placement of a PCIS terminal plus electronic mail capability; and (3) PCIS, electronic mail, and data transfer from the PCIS to the physician's office system and back again.

In stage 3, *data transfer* refers to the exchange of information between the physician's office practice system and the hospital PCIS. These data include test results, clinical notes, and patient schedule information. For example, this data transfer would allow the physician to discharge a hospital patient, transfer a copy of the discharge summary to his or her office computer system, and schedule the patient's next office appointment, all from the hospital PCIS terminal. In terms of time and effort, the savings for both the patient and the physician would be substantial.

The products necessary to achieve all three stages of functionality are currently available. The choices of how much to offer initially and how fast to progress up the ladder are, of course, dependent on resources and demand. In many settings a slow progression is necessary to allow the evolutionary process of education for both physicians and administration to occur. As in the hospital-based PCIS setting, the maximum benefits of the PCIS–office link are obtained when the medical professional both understands and effectively uses the system.

Security

Security (discussed in chapter 6) is essential to the health of any PCIS. However, the special requirements of remote linkages to a PCIS provide special security challenges with respect to the physician's office staff.

In most institutions, in the process of obtaining practice privileges, physicians agree contractually to maintain the confidentiality of patient information and report breaches of security. Therefore, the connection between the PCIS and the physician's office can be viewed as simply an extension of that contract. On the other hand, no contract usually exists between the hospital and the physicians' office employees.

Clearly, such a contract must be drawn up and agreed to, with the medical staff physician as the guarantor. It is also essential that special PCIS pathways be designed for office personnel so that information on only that office's patients is available for viewing. Furthermore, the medical staff and the hospital administration need to discuss, understand, and reach a consensus on the handling of physician office staff security.

Cost

The cost of the PCIS–office links depends on many issues, including the scope of the product being offered, the number of offices to be included, whether those offices are connected by cable or telephone modem, and so on. The cost of the implementation process must also include the type of support system the institution needs. For example, the linkage process may be thought of as simply an extension of the current in-hospital PCIS project, requiring little more than additional equipment and cabling.

Unfortunately, when competitive agendas create a pull between the maintenance of the hospital information system and that of the physician office links, support for the office links might suffer. For example, if the pool of support personnel for hospital information systems is the same as that for physician office systems, when in-hospital systems fail or require emergent attention, service to outlying physician office systems may be severely compromised or discontinued altogether.

In addition, the process of training physician office personnel can place a burden on the resources of the in-hospital PCIS project. If the system is popular and successful, this burden becomes severe, for the training process must take place in many offices.

To handle the training and support requirements for a successful PCIS–office link, service and support personnel from outside the institution can be enlisted to implement the project. For example, an independent office computing service may be employed for all physician office support services, thereby avoiding the problems of competition for in-house support resources.

Another solution is to organize a subsidiary of the hospital to deal with the special needs of the PCIS–office link as well as provide other technology services to physicians' offices, such as facsimile (fax) capabilities and office automation. A for-profit business can be developed by a health care corporation with the defined purpose of physician office automation and technology support. This dedicated business could design and develop physician office systems and implement technology solutions specific to office practice needs (for example, electronic billing and office record keeping).

Summary

Linkages between the PCIS and physicians' offices provide important opportunities to extend the value of the entire system as well as realize new benefits for both the hospital and the medical staff. This chapter has identified the advantages of such linkages and discussed the central considerations for implementing them. The next chapter elaborates on the discussion of the special security demands of a PCIS.

Chapter Six

System Security

Security for the PCIS can be divided into three significant parts: (1) hardware security; (2) software security; and (3) warmware security.

Hardware Security

Hardware security is defined as the stability and reliability of the computers, connections, and other associated equipment in relationship to the requirements of a PCIS. The PCIS places far greater demands on computer hardware than do other standard computer applications, such as financial and clerical systems. In order to provide a reliable link between patient care areas, PCIS hardware must be available 24 hours a day, 365 days a year, and must be up and running from the user's standpoint all of that time. To the extent that the PCIS hardware meets this standard, health care workers come to rely on and use systems as their primary means of communication and documentation of patient care activities. To the extent that the PCIS hardware does not meet these standards, health care workers will retain duplicate systems (such as paper notes and records) and consider the computer system as a secondary, less reliable communication system.

The necessary change in operation of information systems departments to meet these standards, and the shift in priorities to maintain system response time and availability, should not be minimized. The insular nature of hospital data processing departments has made it all too easy for their staffs to consider system availability and response issues as guidelines and recommendations rather than mandatory needs for effective operation. The ethic of information systems departments as true service departments must be recultivated in departments that have come to operate almost autonomously. In addition, if indeed the PCIS hardware security mandate is internalized in an information systems department, necessary considerations such as uninterruptable power supplies and database backup procedures become a natural part of departmental operation.

Special hardware security considerations are operative for physician office connections (as discussed in chapter 5) and for certain terminal locations in which PCIS access must be controlled. With regard to PCIS connections with physicians' offices, the office staff must be trained and given special system passwords if the connections are to work effectively. Because office staff personnel usually have full access to their employing physician's office records, office staff passwords should support access only to those patients cared for by that office's physician.

With regard to PCIS access at other locations, the health care organization needs to consider the special security needs of offering clinicians remote access to a PCIS when they are away from their offices. Telephone/modem access systems that call the user back at a specific location decrease, but do not eliminate, concerns of unauthorized remote access. Continued work on the support technologies is needed to reach the ultimate goal of remote PCIS access, that is, the connection of authorized users to information anywhere.

Terminal location security is the capability of limiting PCIS information access based on the physical location of a terminal. For example, access to psychiatry inpatients is allowed only from terminals on the psychiatry nursing unit. This approach to hardware security can work extremely well for some health care workers, such as nurses, and yet not at all for physicians.

Software Security

Software security is defined as all programming and other operational aspects of the PCIS that perform the following functions:

- Maintain system data integrity
- Provide access control, that is, allow access to patient information only to those intended to have access
- Permit assignment of special security controls to particular data identified by the user as requiring augmented security

Maintenance of PCIS Data Integrity

Maintenance of PCIS data integrity is defined as the stability and inviolability of information entered into a PCIS. For example, if a patient's serum creatinine level is recorded today as 2.5, upon reviewing the electronic record in 10 years the value remains 2.5. Furthermore, system design makes it impossible to alter information added to the electronic patient record, simply to make amendments to it. Without these structures in place, the PCIS cannot act as the primary source of patient information and documentation. In order to successfully manage patient quality of care and risk management issues, these software security control structures must be in place before a PCIS is introduced into a health care system.

Access Control

Access control includes any and all software structures that permit authorized access to patient information and prohibit unauthorized access. Two possible mechanisms of software access control are the electronic signature and PCIS pathway design.

The Electronic Signature

The *electronic signature* is a method of PCIS software security that identifies the users, indelibly stamps all on-line activities with that individual's legal signature, and presents information to the user customized for that particular level of access and job description. In addition, the electronic signature permits on-line order writing and documentation stamped with a clinician's legal signature.

It is essential to inform the user that the convenience and power of the electronic signature comes with a price: individual responsibility. A direct analogy could be made to the automated teller machine (ATM) system that has revolutionized banking. Just as the physician would never pay a debt by giving someone his or her ATM card, the physician user of a PCIS must never share his or her electronic signature. The distribution of this responsibility to all physician users is the cornerstone of true PCIS security.

When physicians request practice privileges at a given institution, they should sign some form of written agreement before receiving access to the PCIS. This agreement ensures the confidentiality of patient information and requires physicians to report any misuse of electronic data. Two sample confidentiality agreements are presented in figures 6-1 and 6-2.

Pathway Design

Pathway design refers to a method of software security that customizes the appearance and operation of a PCIS on the basis of what the user is authorized to do or see and what that user needs to know to do his or her job. For physicians, this could operate as follows: Orthopedic surgeons would automatically be recognized by the system at sign-on and be presented with orthopedic patients and access to common laboratory, radiographic, and surgical resources pertaining to their specialty. They could also access medical patients for consultation, but would not have authorized access to psychiatric inpatients without special password clearance. This security by software design would be easily accepted by users because they are presented with an individualized system at the same time that some access limitations are imposed.

Figure 6-1. Sample Confidentiality Agreement from "Memorial Hospital"

Memorial Hospital
Medical Staff Access Code Confidentiality Agreement

The Patient Care Information System (PCIS) is a medical communication system allowing you to retrieve patient information and enter orders. This document will serve to assure the hospital that you are fully aware of the implications of computer access and the confidentiality involved.

Your utilization of the automated system will communicate information to all users more efficiently and effectively, leading to quality improvement in patient care.

The following statements will provide an understanding of the major significance of the receipt of an access code:

1. I understand that my access code is the equivalent of my legal signature, and I will be accountable for all work done under this code.

2. I understand that the electronic data stored in the PCIS are confidential patient data and must be treated with the same medical–legal care as data in the paper chart.

3. I will not disclose my access code to anyone, nor will I attempt to learn another person's access code.

4. I will not access data on patients for whom I have no responsibilities and for whom I have no "need to know."

5. If I have reason to believe that the confidentiality of my access code has been broken, I will contact Hospital Information Systems Technical Support to have my code changed and a new code issued.

6. I understand that any misuse of my confidential access code will be a violation of Medical Staff policy and could subject me to disciplinary action.

Your signature below acknowledges agreement with these statements.

_____   _____
Name (please print)   Signature

_____
Date

Routing: Information System Data Administration
             Medical Staff
             Medical Staff Office

Figure 6-2. Sample Sign-On Authorization Request from "Community Hospital"

Community Hospital
Hospital Information Services Sign-on Authorization Request

Check one of the following:

_____ Initial request _____ Update _____ Delete _____
Effective date

User's name: _____ _____ _____
Last First Initial

Sign-on ID: _____

Please fill in all of the following information for initial requests. For update requests, fill in only information that has changed.

Name (new): _____

Department: _____ Phone #: _____

Mailing address: Bldg.: _____ Room: _____ Box #: _____

Job title: _____

Social security #: _____ E-mail printer ID: _____

Special requests/comments: _____

Community Hospital has adopted the following policies and procedures to ensure system security and the confidentiality of patient data:

1. System users are responsible for their passwords, and must change them immediately after receiving them.
2. Community Hospital will take disciplinary actions, including dismissal, against anyone who permits:
   - The improper use of his/her sign-on ID
   - The inappropriate dissemination of confidential information

I understand that I am responsible for ensuring that the use of my password conforms to Community Hospital policies and procedures.

User's signature: _____ Date: _____

This ID is needed for the employee to perform his/her duties. This employee is authorized to use available transactions and Master screens. This employee will complete a training class.

Authorized signer: _____ Date: _____

    For HIS use only

Security codes: _____

    Sign-on ID: _____ Password: _____

    Operator ID: _____ Dept. code: _____ Path. flag: _____

    Completed by: _____ Date: _____

Return to: Security Administrator, HIS
Questions: Contact HIS Security

Special Security Controls

Special security controls are best defined by describing their operation. For example, Mrs. Jones, the wife of a prominent member of the medical staff, is admitted to the hospital with a suspicion of acute leukemia. The patient and her husband would like to keep all communication as private as possible between themselves and their physician, Dr. Smith. Dr. Smith signs on to the PCIS and indicates that all aspects of Mrs. Jones's on-line information are "level-1 security," meaning that he personally must authorize any on-line access of her reports and findings. In addition, Mrs. Jones, like every other patient, is provided with a list of the clinicians who have accessed her files during her hospitalization. By this example, it can be seen that special security controls are actually "security on the fly."

Although this type of security capability is often requested, the matter engenders many questions regarding ownership of the PCIS information. For example, how will Dr. Smith control access to Mrs. Jones's information for the hematology laboratory technician who must compare her current blood count with previous values? Special security controls can thus create conflicts between perceived security needs and a user's need to know information to complete his or her particular patient care responsibilities.

Warmware Security

Warmware security pertains to all aspects of PCIS security related to the human use of information. The confidentiality of patient information is the central issue and is clearly not under the control of system hardware design, nor can it be controlled by the operation of software. Instead, the most effective means of ensuring confidentiality is the education of the user. The normal structures for continuing education can be used to prevent or, if necessary, to identify and correct problems among staff in this regard. It is true that PCIS design normally allows for an easy audit of all users' on-line activities, but clearly neither hardware nor software can replace a sound, ongoing effort to educate users on how to protect the confidentiality of patient information.

Lessons in System Security

The importance of system security and user education may be illustrated by the examples of two institutions. One is a university medical center that adopted a simple procedure to address concerns regarding patient confidentiality. The other is a metropolitan medical center that instituted a practice to ensure suitable training for all members of its medical staff.

Instituting an Audit Trail

The trade-offs between access to clinical information needed for patient care and the security of patient information were of serious concern to one university medical center. To address this concern, the institution utilized a feature of its PCIS that could generate a complete audit trail of the information read by physicians as well as the information entered into the system, all identified by electronic signature. The medical staff decided to use this audit trail to print out a report of all the physicians who have viewed a patient's electronic medical record during hospitalization.

The report is provided to the patient at the time of discharge. This practice was publicized widely within the institution to all attending and resident staff. The response from both medical staff and patients has been unanimously positive.

Ensuring thorough Intern Training

The experience of a second institution illustrates the importance of the commitment to security by all members of the medical staff. At this metropolitan medical center, a medical intern failed to attend proficiency training on the institution's PCIS before beginning his clinical rotation. Although his supervising resident offered to enter the evening's orders into the PCIS for the intern "just this once," the intern "borrowed" the resident's electronic signature and wrote orders on all patients that evening. This was reported by the supervising resident to PCIS security administration the next day. The information was then relayed to the medical director of the residency training program.

The intern was given the choice of completing his PCIS training within the next 24 hours or being dismissed from the program. He chose the latter. The medical director of the residency training program treated the intern's behavior as the serious breach of security and professional conduct that it was. This event was widely discussed among the medical staff, as well as the residents and the interns. Current practice at this institution is such that interns would no more begin their clinical duties without a PCIS electronic signature than write prescriptions without a valid medical license.

Summary

PCIS security must take into account not only hardware and software, but warmware as well. There is no better source of security than the user who is educated in PCIS functions and behaves responsibly. Therefore, the ongoing maintenance of system security requires a concerted effort on the part of both users and system personnel to be effective. Security also requires an ongoing dedication of the physician task force to keep up to date with system security issues and to keep these issues in the forefront of discussions among the medical staff.

Chapter Seven

System Benefits and Evaluation

The previous chapters have begun to reveal the unique benefits that a PCIS can offer to a health care organization and its medical staff and patients. This chapter further explores the benefits realized when physicians collaborate on the selection, design, and implementation of a PCIS. It also explains how to measure and monitor those benefits.

Chapter 1 discussed the important aspects of direct physician involvement in, and use of, a PCIS. The case was made that even if a PCIS is installed with the expectation of improving the quality of patient care, and even if physicians are the primary decision makers in setting patient care plans and using health care resources, the benefits of having a PCIS will only be fully realized if physicians directly use the information tools in their day-to-day clinical decision-making and patient care activities.

The realms of clinical computing and hospital information systems have been on parallel tracks for some time. On the one hand, clinical computing, medical informatics, and other physician-directed information technology efforts have evolved along clinically specific lines, usually under the umbrella of applied research. Projects have yielded significant breakthroughs in primary research, medical education, and artificial intelligence applications, but have rarely taken on the challenge of full automation of hospitals, clinics, and the business of patient care. On the other hand, HCISs have been limited to the financial and clerical aspects of computing, thereby giving only minimal consideration to the essential aspects of clinical decision making (such as the accommodation of DRGs into system functionality).

In the current climate of financial constraints and regulation, the continued support and the unfettered development of both the clinical and financial/clerical tracks are most unlikely. Therefore, a forced marriage of sorts between these two directions in health care computing development is necessary. The reality of achieving maximal financial benefits from clinical information systems will be exacted by potential hospital buyers, and the clinical utility and patient care value of hospital information systems will be scrutinized by medical staffs participating in PCIS purchasing decisions.

Therefore, a unique benefit of a PCIS project that directly involves physicians is the increased likelihood of fulfilling both the clinical and institutional goals of that project.

Monitoring Physician Utilization of the Information System

Because some of the primary benefits of the PCIS are directly related to the degree of utilization by physicians, some objective instrument must be derived to serve as a report card for the physician training effort. For example, consider the PCIS utilization report shown in figure 7-1. This report may be designed by information systems programmers to provide monthly or annual reports of direct physician use of the PCIS.

As discussed in chapter 1, the sine qua non of physician use of the PCIS is order writing. The physician utilization report in figure 7-1 tallies all orders entered into the PCIS each month by or for each physician, and specifies what percentage of the orders was entered by the physician and what percentage by an agent for the physician (such as a nurse, a ward clerk, or a technical staff member). The report also provides percentages detailing the kinds of orders entered by the agent for the physician, that is, verbal, written, or protocol orders:

- *Verbal orders* are those orders given orally by the physician to the agent. The use of this form of order is usually limited to emergency situations and in the operating, emergency, and critical care areas.
- *Written orders* are those orders written by the physician and transcribed into the PCIS by the agent for the physician. Obviously, those physicians not certified to use the PCIS will continue to use written orders.
- *Protocol orders* are orders entered for the physician by specialized personnel according to protocol. For example, nurse practitioners, nurse midwives, and physician assistants all may enter orders for a physician according to predefined medical staff protocols.

Figure 7-1. Sample PCIS Physician Utilization Summary Report

Physician Name	Total # Orders	Orders Entered by Physician	Orders Entered by Agent	Verbal Orders	Written Orders	Protocol Orders
Bill Bria	501	80%	20%	15%	3%	2%
John Smith	720	20%	80%	40%	15%	25%
Jeff Jones	436	5%	95%	10%	85%	0%

If printed monthly, this summary report of physician utilization can provide important system management information. As illustrated in figure 7-1, Dr. Bria is a typical PCIS user, who personally enters 80 percent of his orders into the system. He works in the intensive care unit, so he occasionally uses verbal orders but almost never resorts to written orders. At first glance, Dr. Smith appears to be a rather poor system user, with only 20 percent of his orders directly entered. However, Dr. Smith works in the emergency room, where verbal and protocol orders are most common. Therefore, a 20-percent direct-order entry is actually quite good for a physician in this clinical setting, and he should be congratulated for his efforts.

Dr. Jones, however, demonstrates a different pattern. Although he is an internist certified to use the PCIS, he still writes out 85 percent of his orders, which others then have to enter into the PCIS for him. This physician clearly has a problem with effectively using the PCIS. A collegial phone call from the medical director of information systems would be in order to help identify the problem(s) Dr. Jones is having with the system and offer personal (and confidential) assistance to help improve his usage and benefit from the PCIS.

The physician utilization report can be useful in a number of ways: (1) to document physician use of the PCIS; (2) to evaluate the success of specific training efforts at increasing individual and group utilization; and (3) to serve as a management tool for the medical director of information systems to help target physicians who need assistance in order to make effective use of the PCIS. Although many factors enter into the percentage of total orders directly entered by physicians, this number is nevertheless valuable for determining the extent to which the system is doing what it was designed to do. That is, it is only when physicians directly use the PCIS that feedback on drug interactions, cost of medications, and the like, is delivered directly to the individuals responsible for the clinical decisions—the physicians themselves.

Assistance with Medical Decision Making

With a true clinically directed PCIS that finds widespread acceptance among the medical staff on a consistent basis, the expected benefits should extend beyond order writing to medical decision making. The following are just some of the possible areas of study for enhancing the effectiveness of a PCIS:

1. Benefits of having essential patient information available at the time of clinical decision making
2. Time and cost savings achieved by having all patient test results, both inpatient and outpatient, immediately available to physicians on-line

3. Impact on ordering practices of providing cost and clinical information to physicians on-line at the moment of ordering a particular high-cost or high-resource-consuming clinical procedure

4. Efficiency of patient "through-put," that is, an examination of the time it takes for patients to get in and out of an outpatient information system *before* versus *after* the implementation of a PCIS

5. Physician time saving and practice efficiency

6. Impact of a PCIS connection to outreach outpatient clinics and physician offices

7. Effect of providing patient, diagnosis, and physician-specific quality assurance (QA) information on-line to physicians at the time of ordering and planning workup strategies

   To illustrate the benefits of a PCIS for medical decision making, imagine a physician entering orders on a 45-year-old male patient diagnosed with acute cholecystitis. Before the physician begins entering orders, she selects *patient QA information.* She is then presented with a report, the product of information collected from national and local medical information databases, showing the effects on clinical outcome of various treatments (for example, surgery, gallstone-dissolving agents, clinical observation alone) on a male patient between the ages of 40 and 50. The outcome information is first presented as the national average, followed by information on the specific experience in the physician's own hospital (from data collected on the PCIS).

   Finally, the physician has the choice of viewing outcomes for similar patients with this diagnosis in her practice as compared with the outcomes for patients of other physicians on staff (with the physicians' names removed for confidentiality). Imagine the profound impact this information, presented in this way through a PCIS, would have on medical decision making and the quality of patient care!

Provision of Quality-Related Information to Physicians

The issue of providing QA information to physicians bears further discussion. For some time now, the process of clinical QA has been a retrospective review of clinical practice defined by screens of clinically important data and issues. The QA reporting process continues in most hospitals in the form of written notices and group presentations to physicians in the hope that practice behavior can be influenced and improved. At best, the influence on physicians lasts for a short time, and then, because specific information is not continually provided to them at the time of clinical decision making, the issue is forgotten.

A PCIS provides an unparalleled opportunity to address all aspects of the clinical QA process: (1) QA screen identification; (2) QA data collection and analysis; and (3) the most effective QA reporting and feedback system possible for influencing clinical decisions.

Screen Identification

The PCIS provides a means of QA screen identification via a review of the vast amount of on-line, day-to-day clinical practice information that it holds. With this large amount of real-time practice information, physicians and others can identify practice trends, important clinical questions and issues, and variations in practice and patient outcomes that could form the best institution-specific QA screens directed toward improving the quality of patient care. Obviously, security of information and review would have to be carefully preserved; however, the availability of hospital-, patient-, diagnosis-, and physician-specific information increases the chances that truly relevant, clinically important QA screens will be developed.

Data Collection and Analysis

It follows that the PCIS would be the most effective QA data collector because system information could be transferred automatically to the special QA database. Once it is confidentially coded, information on all clinically relevant cases could be identified and analyzed.

The parallel to clinical research is obvious, because using a PCIS for QA screen identification is, in fact, a form of clinical research case finding. It is only too clear that the scope of all medical issues deserving formal study is far beyond the capabilities of traditional research methods, in terms of both labor and cost. With effective PCISs, however, each clinical center has a tool for regular, cost-effective clinical study, with the added benefit that the results can be extremely specific and relevant to the patient and practitioner community.

Reporting and Feedback

Following data collection and analysis, the PCIS could provide its strongest QA benefit to the hospital community in the form of on-line reporting and feedback to specific physicians. Clearly, the PCIS could be used for on-line copies of the latest QA reports for physician review. However, the QA benefits would be even greater if the feedback were made context-sensitive and at the clinically appropriate moment.

For example, it is somewhat effective, and hence arguably useful, to inform physicians upon sign-on to a PCIS that a recent QA study has shown greater use of a particularly expensive antibiotic than would be expected for that hospital and its patient population. However, it is clearly far more powerful for the PCIS to present a specific list of antibiotics to the physician for order selection, all of which would be effective against the bacteria cultured in the microbiology laboratory on that particular patient, in order of cost per dose. Such a context-sensitive, timely response demonstrates the ability of a PCIS to be utilized as a smart method for QA information feedback, thereby enabling the hospital to reap the maximum benefits of a QA process.

Case Study

To better illustrate how to study the impact of a PCIS on medical decision making, consider the following example. Before completing PCIS implementation, the medical staff at hospital B wished to investigate the real impact on clinical practice of having a PCIS. A study group was formed and eventually developed a hypothesis: If the PCIS is a permanent electronic medical record, and if the PCIS will instantly present medical information and history required by the physician for medical decision making, the PCIS will be the preferred information tool by physicians in daily medical practice.

The group reasoned that one of the best areas in the hospital to demonstrate the benefits of the PCIS would be the emergency ward (EW), where there are defined time limitations on clinical decision making. The group also felt that EW physicians would be able to quickly rank the relative value of all the available sources of patient information. In doing so, the PCIS would be compared with three other patient information instruments also available in the EW: (1) the previous EW visit records kept in the EW for two months following the last visit; (2) the patient's last hospitalization discharge summary, faxed to the EW by the medical records department; and (3) the complete written medical record.

Each EW physician was asked to fill out one evaluation sheet for each of the four information instruments used. Because it was clear that all portions of the written medical record would not be of equal value in the process of medical decision making, each physician was also asked to rank the information instruments by the type of clinical information (for example, discharge instructions, lab tests, medical history, and so forth). Figure 7-2 is an example of an evaluation sheet similar to the one used in this investigation.

The type of study used by hospital B requires minimal cost and development time, yet results in an objective demonstration of the benefits of a PCIS. The data obtained from such an investigation can also be used to identify deficiencies in the PCIS and establish priorities for further development.

Figure 7-2. Medical Record Utilization Study

Diagnosis: _____

Information retrieved from: (Please circle one.)

PCIS   Previous EW Record   Faxed Discharge   Patient's Complete
        within 2 Months   Summary   Record

Usefulness to Emergency Ward Evaluation Treatment and Disposition
(Please check appropriate category.)

Type of Information	Reviewed, But Not Necessary	Interesting, But Not Necessary	Helpful and Necessary	Critical to Patient Care
Demographic information	[ ]	[ ]	[ ]	[ ]
Patient visit history (# of visits to EW)	[ ]	[ ]	[ ]	[ ]
Physician who saw patient	[ ]	[ ]	[ ]	[ ]
Medical history	[ ]	[ ]	[ ]	[ ]
Physician exams	[ ]	[ ]	[ ]	[ ]
Lab tests	[ ]	[ ]	[ ]	[ ]
EKGs	[ ]	[ ]	[ ]	[ ]
Other tests	[ ]	[ ]	[ ]	[ ]
Hospital course	[ ]	[ ]	[ ]	[ ]
Medication history	[ ]	[ ]	[ ]	[ ]
Discharge instructions	[ ]	[ ]	[ ]	[ ]
Patient's discharge diagnosis	[ ]	[ ]	[ ]	[ ]

Documentation and Other Benefits

One of the greatest burdens on modern medicine is the increasing demand for documentation of care. Numerous groups, including peer review organizations, the Joint Commission on Accreditation of Healthcare Organizations, insurance companies, home care agencies, and so forth, all require specific clinical information. The generation of that information results in extra responsibilities and writing time for nurses, physicians, and other health care providers. It has been estimated that nurses spend over 40 percent of their time tending to these documentation requirements. Therefore, one of the most important benefits of a clinically directed PCIS is that it provides a means of decreasing time spent in documentation. A computer's ability to bring together any element in its data bank and reformat the output in essentially any manner makes even the most Spartan PCIS deliver on this important benefit.

For example, the list of a patient's active medications is important to essentially all individuals who have to participate in that patient's clinical management (including those who have to rate the patient's level of care). A PCIS would automatically maintain this list because the PCIS is the primary ordering tool for retaining and transmitting the order in the first place. Active orders can then be presented in many ways: by category (for example, antibiotics, sedatives), by route of administration (for example, intravenous or oral medications), by diagnosis (for example, oncologic agents), or even by cost. Any authorized user can have his or her own copy of the information, in the appropriate format, for the asking. The time saved by decreasing the current demands of documentation may, of course, be used in many ways. It is obviously up to the individual whether that extra time is spent with the patient or elsewhere.

Summary

The implementation of a PCIS provides an institution with the opportunity to examine all aspects of an organization's operation and delivery of patient care. As this book has demonstrated, the automation of all aspects of clinical practice requires data collection, data analysis, and thorough implementation of PCIS functionality. Therefore, this three-part process affords an institution an unequaled opportunity to change the existing "dogma" and inefficiencies propagated for no other reason than, to quote an often-heard phrase, "That's the way we do it here."

The process of introducing a clinically driven PCIS often identifies opportunities for cost and time savings as well as brings many clinical practices up to date. For example, hospital patient registration activities may presently be collecting a large amount of underused information, thereby slowing down the patient care process while failing to collect important data relative to lines of referral, new patterns of disease treatment, and the general use of hospital resources. Implementation of a PCIS gives the health care organization an opportunity to enhance and streamline operations. If physicians are involved, clinical as well as operational changes can be identified and implemented for the betterment of both the organization and its patients.

Chapter Eight

Dealing with Managed Care: A Strategic Model for Clinical Information

These are uncertain times in U.S. medicine. The debate over managed care has accelerated the rate at which health care is changing but leaves many wondering about the impact of this rapid change on medical education, research, and indigent care. Certainly managed care in the United States is now more clearly focused on financial opportunities in the absence of any controlling federal legislation, allowing it to grow according to existing market forces.

Managed care will also have a profound effect on the physician–computer connection. In posing the question, "Will managed care negatively or positively affect the physician–computer connection?," we believe the answer is an unequivocal "Yes!" The reasons for this ambivalent response are as follows.

Managed care is predicated on the availability of reliable data about the financial performance of any health care entity, be it a physician, hospital, network of hospitals, or regional health care system. It is upon this information that the fundamental assumptions for developing a managed care enterprise can be based, and upon which certain entities and individuals are included or excluded. However, because health care financial information is more available than clinical information, the connection between clinical decision making and financial data still eludes most health care systems.

Another tenet of managed care is the need to change physician behavior. Because physicians dictate over 80 percent of the allocation of health care resources, and because managed care is dedicated to both limiting costs and distributing resources in the most effective and efficient way possible, an information link is needed between the care management and the ordering physician. With such a link, the managed care process actually will facilitate the physician–computer connection. The reason is that, to achieve the physician-ordering behavior modification that most managed care programs seek, a real-time process that allows physicians to consider the patient's needs and the system's cost requirements is needed. The best way to achieve this "just-in-time" aspect of the clinical decision-making process is for the physician to use a computer as his or her order communication instrument.

The Need for Clinical Information

Support for the managed care benefits of promoting the physician–computer connection appear in a recently published meta-analysis of the clinical decision support (CDS) literature.[1] There is an additional positive element to the relationship between the physician–computer connection and managed care: financial success. Physicians are becoming involved in self-managing new managed care entities—for example, physician health care organizations (PHOs). To provide the kind of management information physicians need to operate these new organizations, a continuing process of data collection at the point of care is necessary. As physicians themselves realize that this is essential to their ongoing success, financial and otherwise, they begin to use clinical information systems (CISs) more successfully. Peer pressure now is financial pressure as well. As a stockholder, the clinician is interested in the success of the managed care business. It may be argued that the transition from a fee-for-service environment to managed and capitated care can actually facilitate change in physicians' daily ordering behavior.

Alternatively it may be argued that the growth of managed care will hinder the physician–computer connection significantly because managed care is squarely focused on the financial bottom line. The cost of installing the necessary information infrastructure (for example, networks, workstations, and software) is substantial. Physicians in many managed care organizations are employees rather than independent contractors. Hence, if the organization wants to modify physician-ordering behavior, it simply needs to identify those physicians who spend the most resources, request them to change their behavior, and reassign them if change does not occur. As long as the financial bottom line is served, the managed care organization could leave all the behavior modification to the individual clinician. Using the current financial information system infrastructure already in place in most hospitals, the managed care organization could continue to monitor the performance of physician employees and reassign those who are practicing at "too high a cost" to the organization. This process would require no new CISs and could still keep costs to a minimum. However, the obvious difficulty with this financial-based system is the lack of meaningful quality information, which can undermine even the most carefully developed financial models. Nevertheless, as illustrated in this scenario, the managed care movement could actually stop the physician–computer connection in its tracks.

Whether or not the physician–computer connection will be accelerated by the change to managed health care in this country is in many ways the same as asking whether we will balance the control of health care costs with improvement in the quality of that care. Because few U.S. medical centers have successfully achieved direct physician connection to their HCISs, we can hope that the realization of the change in physician behavior will be most closely coupled with an understanding of quality information for patient care. Only through methods that improve this connection will lasting changes be made in physician-ordering behavior.

A Three-Dimensional Model for Clinical Information

With the failure of Congress to pass managed care legislation, some have suggested that this country can now take its time in considering the best way to proceed with health care change. However, it is obvious that change in U.S. health care is occurring rapidly without any further federal legislation. Nevertheless, the changes are occurring more at a regional level than on a national scale. That fact has the following implications for physicians:

- Because an organized national plan has not been formulated, market forces will likely play the predominant role in the speed and nature of the change to managed care.
- The pace of regional change will not be predictable. Without a national coordinated program, business forces have driven change literally overnight, making adaptation especially challenging.
- Although the national health care reform legislation *did* take medical education into account, most business and financially motivated regional health care reform programs do not. Therefore, there may be significant risk to continued support for the higher overhead costs incurred by medical education programs.

With the growth of regional managed care, most health care organizations are now planning or implementing regional health care networks consisting of interinstitutional agreements, practice purchases and consolidations, and expanded ambulatory care facilities. Concomitantly there has been an interest in a new form of information infrastructure, the community health information network (CHIN), which has enabled technology to meet the challenge of constructing these new health care environments.

To make sense of the current panoply of information structures and systems, a CIS model is needed. There are three advantages to using an overall strategic model:

- The critical building blocks of a comprehensive information system strategy can be identified and laid out.
- The critical interrelationships of the components can be described and understood.
- A process for using clinical information, with one part of the cycle leading to another, can be best visualized and described.

Without a demonstration of what a complete, enterprisewide CIS model is, one can become quickly lost in a sea of acronyms, jargon, and unrealistic expectations.

Figure 8-1 presents a three-dimensional model for a CIS. The model can easily be visualized with the Cartesian coordinate system showing the X, Y, and Z axes describing the location of objects in three-dimensional space.

Figure 8-1.   A Three-Dimensional Health Care Enterprise Model for a CIS

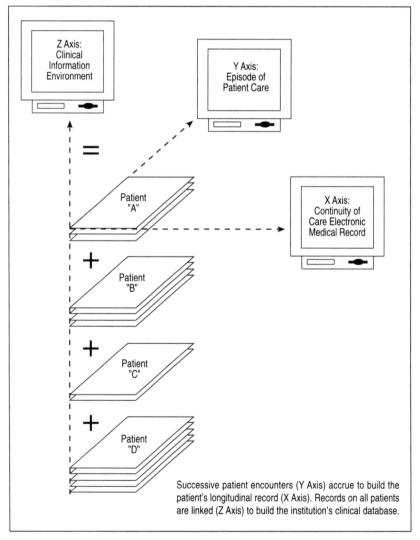

Successive patient encounters (Y Axis) accrue to build the patient's longitudinal record (X Axis). Records on all patients are linked (Z Axis) to build the institution's clinical database.

The Y Axis: An Episode of Patient Care

The Y axis represents an episode of patient care. This episode may be a single point in time, such as a hospital admission, a one-time office visit, or an emergency department visit. It can also represent a recurring visit for a specific clinical purpose that constitutes one episode. For example, one logical episode of care could be a visit to a coumadin therapy clinic, the sole purpose of which is the maintenance of the proper level of the anticoagulant.

Within the context of a patient care episode, the Y axis of our CIS model possesses the following characteristics:

- Integration of patient information: All information on the individual patient (demographics, diagnoses, medications, allergies, insurance, and so forth) is brought forward around the decision making necessary within the single episode of care.
- Integration of decision support information: This is just-in-time medical decision support. Here the prior authorization for services from a managed care plan, as well as the clinical guideline for improving the quality of care and the specific cost information relative to all available alternatives for care, are brought together to help the health care worker make an appropriate decision.
- Rapid operation: The Y axis of our model is an information tool to be used on a daily basis for the communication of actual results and orders. Thus, a key characteristic is speed. Rapid operation is critical for acceptance of any information tool into daily clinical practice.[2]
- Clinically intuitive information presentation: It is possible to present so much information that the clinical user is overwhelmed and the information goes unprocessed and unused. Over many years, a clinician develops a methodology to deal with the large amounts of information that have become a daily part of clinical practice. If that methodology is used in the design of the Y axis of a CIS, then the clinician can navigate the information successfully and will "drill down" to details of that information database as needed. Otherwise the tour de force of presenting all relevant information on a patient during an episode of care is just that—only a technical achievement and not really of benefit to the process of clinical decision making. This characteristic of "clinical intuitiveness" is far more complex and elusive than the example implies. Although the aforementioned CIS methodology is consistent within a medical discipline, such as internal medicine, there are important variations between disciplines (surgery, ob/gyn, pediatrics, and so on) and even more significant variations between other clinical professions (for example, nursing, allied health care workers, and so forth). Hence the breadth and depth of this component of the Y axis is challenging to even the most flexible and well-designed

CIS environment. This is one of the reasons that CIS development and refinement is an iterative process.

The X Axis: The Continuity of Care Electronic Record

The X axis of our model may be described as the compilation of every one of the Y axis episodes of care, placed one next to the other. All the episodes of care of an individual patient amount to the continuity of care electronic medical record. This record would logically follow the patient wherever he or she sought medical care, thereby making the X axis a permanent "birth-to-death" patient record. Again, this portion of our CIS model has the following distinct characteristics:

- Comprehensiveness: Obviously if the electronic birth-to-death medical record fails to include important elements of that individual's medical history, it will cease to be the authoritative source of information on that patient. On the other hand, unless an individual has had all his or her medical care rendered in a single medical center (increasingly unlikely in the United States), then essentially neither paper nor electronic records truly meet this requirement. In the growing era of CHINs, however, this characteristic may more likely be present in the years to come.
- Structure: With the capability of holding large amounts of clinical, financial, and other information, if that information is without an "index," a table of contents, or some other recognizable structure that allows easy navigation through it, the X axis will be only so much electronic noise. This structure will need to be either entered into the record during its creation (unlikely, given the failure of a uniform medical language and record structure after hundreds of years of medical practice) or imposed on the existing information after entry.
- Intelligence: The electronic record must also contain some built-in intelligence if it is to truly augment clinicians' ability to manage ambulatory care in a logical and timely manner. Specifically, the record must possess the intelligence to notify the clinician when crucial health maintenance situations arise (such as the need for mammography in a patient with a family history of breast cancer). Also the X axis continuity system must allow intelligent information retrieval (such as the ability to respond to a request to "please display the last abnormal chest X ray").

The Z Axis: The Clinical Information Environment

The Z axis represents the dimension of CIS that is universally desired: the ability to navigate information across patients across time or episodes of care. It is here in the Z axis that the true benefit of collecting information from the other two dimensions begins to be realized. Queries such as, "Show me all patients I have cared for who have developed renal insufficiency on NSAIDs," and "How soon do my acute asthma patients return to work as compared with my colleagues' patients?" can be answered. This information dimension also defines the space for clinical research and investigation. Indeed this Z axis provides the potential for turning every health care organization into its own ongoing prospective research environment, providing specific information on the collective experience of all patients and providers at a particular location. This latter feature is becoming more important as CHINs stretch across the country highlighting differences and similarities between patient groups. The Z axis is also the health care planning data repository, providing a "data-based" management of our health care resources in a more intelligent, patient- and region-specific way than was ever before possible.

The characteristics of this CIS dimension are as follows:

- Flexibility: By the nature of the example queries listed above, it should be evident to the reader that this information dimension requires a very flexible structure allowing a very broad range of reports to be solicited, the majority of which may not be specifically known prior to the collection of the supporting information base. Natural language query structures would be of significant value in this Z dimension. For example, the request, "Find the patients who have had a liver transplant and who have returned to work," yields a list of postsurgery patients who have achieved this important outcome.
- Comprehensiveness: Unlike the narrow specificity needed for the Y and X axes when seeking information on an individual patient, this axis demands a complete organized database that reveals relationships between patients, providers, therapies, and so on that can be appreciated only if all relevant information is contained.
- Agility: The Z axis clinical information environment must provide the ability to meet new business needs of the extremely volatile and mutating health care environment in this country. Because reporting requirements and regulations may lag far behind actual need for strategic information to all health care organizations and workers to best adapt to these changing times, so must the information environment supporting their efforts adjust and adapt to those needs.

Completing the Cycle of Clinical Information

If the three dimensions of the CIS model are viewed as separate and distinct elements on the Cartesian axes, then the most important dimension of interrelationships would not be realized. Rather we view the Y, X, and Z axes as a cycle of information, much as figure 8-2 describes their relationships.

Figure 8-2. The Cycle of CIS

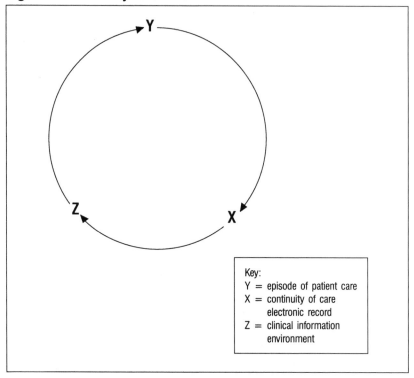

Key:
Y = episode of patient care
X = continuity of care
     electronic record
Z = clinical information
     environment

It is rather easy to envision the flow of information from the Y axis (the vertically integrated view) to the X axis (the continuity of care record). Likewise it is logical to understand that the collected repository of each patient's X axis (permanent patient record) creates the basis for the relational information tool that is the Z axis. However, the knowledge obtained via access to the Z axis – the ability to construct practice guidelines, care maps, and other structures based on true outcome need for patients within a particular practice or health care system by closing the last portion of the loop, the Z to Y axes – could have a truly remarkable effect on our health care system. It is this element of the CIS model that will be discussed further.

All existing quality of care methods to date have depended on retrospective information for initial problem identification. Once new knowledge was gained, it was provided in a retrospective manner, eliciting more defensiveness from clinicians than cooperation. By closing the three-dimensional CIS information loop, we can achieve true prospective quality improvement via an entirely new process, just-in-time CDS. This type of CDS system would allow the practitioner to have the full benefit of a new clinical guideline, itself identified and developed out of the experience within that practitioner's own health care environment, and include that information at the moment of the next ordering decision. This new prospective, relevant, databased CDS system has the full capability of truly improving the quality of care of *every* patient cared for using this information environment. In fact, this promise is already beginning to be realized at several forward-thinking medical centers, including LDS Hospital in Salt Lake City, and the Brigham and Women's Hospital in Boston.[3] The topic of CDS is treated more fully in chapter 9.

Summary

This chapter presented a three-dimensional strategic model for CISs that takes into account the important data needed in a managed care environment. Armed with the right information, the practitioner can approach the design and/or selection of CISs from a broader managed care information perspective, and improve the likelihood that the necessary clinical information needed to meet the challenges of managed care will be available where and when necessary.

References

1. Johnston, M. E., Langton, K. B., Haynes, R. B., and Mathieu, A. Effects of computer-based clinical decision support systems on clinician performance and outcome: a critical appraisal of research. *Annals of Internal Medicine* 120(2):134–42, Jan. 15, 1994.

2. Gall, J. E., Norwood, D. D., Cook, M., Fleming, J. F., Rydell, R., and Watson, R. J. *Demonstration and Evaluation of a Total Hospital Information System.* NCHSR Research Summary Series. U.S. Department of Health, Education and Welfare Public Health Service, Health Resources Administration, HRA77-3188, July 1977.

3. Evans, R. S., Classen, D. C., Pestotnik, S. L., Lundsgaarde, H. P., and Burke, J. P. Improving empiric antibiotic selection using computer decision support. *Archives of Internal Medicine* 154(8):878–84, Apr. 25, 1994.

Chapter Nine

Clinical Decision Support and the Future of U.S. Health Care

In a milestone article in the *Journal of the American Medical Informatics Association,* William Stead, MD, and Dean Sittig outlined the following demonstrable benefits of physician order entry:[1]

- Process improvement
- Cost-effective decision making
- Efficient use of clinician time
- CDS

This chapter discusses three of those benefits and describes the experience of two organizations in realizing such benefits.

Process Improvement

Process improvement pertains to the improved communication, documentation, and efficiencies of a fully integrated direct physician order-entry system. For example, when the physician orders a radiology test to be performed, nursing and radiology are simultaneously and immediately notified of the request. Dietary also is automatically notified as to the change in diet to best complete the radiology exam. The order itself is electronically added to the day's order list and to the nursing, dietary, and radiology worklists. Physician order entry thus facilitates the routine communications of patient care and is a substantial improvement over even the most effective traditional systems.

Cost-Effective Decision Making

The ability of computer-aided decision support systems to improve cost-effective decision making has been well documented in the literature.[2] When clinicians are presented with both clinical information and cost information, they will consistently strive to make the most effective *and* most cost-effective choices.[3] Hence, a direct physician order communication system can present cost-of-care information "just in time," permitting an informed cost-effective decision process to occur.

Clinical Decision Support

Another demonstrable benefit of a direct physician order communication system is CDS, an essential element of the three-dimensional CIS model discussed in chapter 8. It may well be the most important benefit to patients, physicians, nurses, and health care systems of a PCIS. It is first important to clearly define what is meant by "clinical decision support."

CDS may be defined as ". . . knowledge systems which use two or more items of patient data to generate case-specific advice."[4] The key element of this definition is "two or more items," implying an information view that brings together the many elements necessary to truly aid clinical decision making and provide "case-specific advice." General clinical information resources, such as Medline, are certainly useful reference resources; however, they are rarely practical for providing *case-specific* clinical information at the moment of clinical decision making. In fact, the only information tool that can provide such rapid, integrated, and case-specific CDS information is the PCIS. With this definition of CDS in mind, what are the data supporting the performance of CDS systems in improving health care outcomes and changing clinician practice behavior?

The Performance of CDS Systems

In 1994, Mary Johnston, MD, and the medical informatics department at McMaster University, Hamilton, Ontario, Canada, reported on the effects of computer-based CDS systems on clinical performance and patient outcomes.[5] This meta-analysis of the existing literature on CDS combed through 793 citations using a variety of criteria largely intended to identify articles in which some element of study controls and methods could be identified. It is interesting that only 28 articles met those criteria for analysis. Johnston and her group divided those 28 articles into five categories:

- Drug-dosing studies
- Computer-aided diagnosis studies
- Preventive care reminder studies
- Computer-aided QA studies
- Patient outcomes studies

Three of the four evaluable drug-dosing studies showed a significant improvement in clinician performance—largely a result of improvement in identification of drug and drug–allergy interactions. The effectiveness of automatic drug interaction and dosing checking has been recognized for many years and in many settings (for example, inpatient, emergency services, and office practice).[6]

Computer-aided diagnosis studies in general failed to show a significant benefit in clinician performance. This finding was confirmed in a 1994 article[7] that reported on the testing of three commercial computer-aided diagnostic programs using standard clinical case scenarios. After case information was entered into each program, even after more than 20 possible different diagnoses were listed by the programs, only 50 percent of the relevant diagnoses for each case were actually listed. The complexity of "artificial intelligence" replication of general clinical diagnosis has been noted in the literature for some time.[8] Targeted specialty-oriented diagnosis support programs have enjoyed a bit more success, although, as a result of their significant information maintenance requirements, they have very limited application and distribution (Mycin, Oncocin). Recently a computer-aided diagnosis system, Knowledge Couplers, has been developed that standardizes the clinical history questions asked and provides a weighted list of diagnoses.[9]

Four out of the six preventive care reminder studies reviewed showed a significant improvement in clinician performance. As U.S. health care services shift focus from inpatient to ambulatory care, this demonstrable benefit of CDS will take on greater importance. In particular, the shift in emphasis from high technology "reparative" health care to preventive health care will benefit from the consistency of computerized reminders in busy outpatient practices.

QA processes are commonly retrospective, in which "compliance" with QA screens is monitored, reported to clinicians, and then remeasured. The logistical ability to present quality information to clinicians just in time at the next resource allocation decision point has long been a frustration for all involved in the QA and total quality improvement processes. In seven of nine studies in which CDS systems were used to concurrently and prospectively remind clinicians of quality standards, the improvement in performance was noted. These studies provide an important starting point for rethinking the methodology of QA and continuous quality improvement health care processes, for if CDS systems significantly improve the actual outcomes of these programs, a new standard of QA implementation could be in the making.

Finally, out of the 10 patient outcomes studies that Johnston and her group analyzed, only 3 were shown to improve patient outcomes. The authors remark, and we quite agree, that this may be an artifact of the very few outcomes studies and the immaturity of outcomes study methodology in the literature rather than a true negative effect of CDS systems. In fact, the many outcomes indicated by the article categories mentioned above would suggest that properly focused outcomes studies should indeed show significant impact on patient outcomes, as they have shown positive change in clinician performance.

Decision Support at LDS Hospital

A recent study by LDS Hospital in Salt Lake City demonstrates the value of case-specific CDS systems in improving physician clinical performance. David Classen, MD, and others at LDS Hospital developed an expert system that was integrated with the hospital's PCIS.[10] Their system collected information on empiric (that is, without definite culture results) antibiotic therapy of common infections at LDS. The database included weighted listings of the most common organisms isolated by diagnosis, the antibiotic sensitivity spectrum of those organisms, and the cost for 24 hours of treatment by each of the relevant antibiotics. The system also suggested an empiric antibiotic to the ordering physician that could be immediately accepted or an alternate drug selected. Patient allergy profiles, renal function, and other factors were automatically included in the expert system's recommendations, as it had access to the entire integrated electronic medical record system.

Dr. Classen and his colleagues performed several important outcome measurements:

- System utilization
- Time to select the antibiotic to which the patient's culture-infecting organisms were sensitive (extremely important both to medical outcome and to time in the hospital)
- Physician satisfaction with the ordering methodology

Classen and his group discovered the following:

- Each ordering physician used the antibiotic CDS system at least three times per day.
- Pre- versus postsystem implementation showed a significant decrease in the time from patient admission to when the proper effective antibiotic was administered.
- Physicians believed the time taken in using the CDS system was well spent and actually improved the care their patients were receiving.

It is hoped that this study is the first of many showing that physicians can effectively use properly implemented, case-specific, integrated CDS systems to improve both the cost effectiveness of health care and the quality of that care.

Building a CDS System at the Brigham and Women's Hospital: A Case Study

The Brigham and Women's Hospital (BWH) in Boston has long been regarded as one of the leading health care institutions in this country. It has also long been considered one of the most aggressive in adopting new technologies in PCISs. The recent success of BWH's new integrated CIS, the Brigham Integrated Computing System (BICS), has been hailed as a modern success story in making the physician–computer connection. In fall 1994, the authors visited BWH to help capture the elements of that success. The importance of a dedicated visionary leader in information systems, such as John P. Glaser, vice-president of information systems and BWH, and physician leaders including John Teich, MD, medical director of computer systems and architect of the order-entry portion of BICS, is clearly demonstrated in this Boston health care system.

Over the past 10 years, BWH has built and rebuilt systems on many platforms: mainframe, minicomputers, and personal computer local area networks. In fact, the BWH system is built entirely on a client/server system consisting of 80 486 Intel chip personal computers. The current BICS consists of an entirely in-house development integrated information system based on the MUMPS (Massachusetts General Hospital Utility Multi Programming System) programming language. MUMPS is an extensible database useful in medical applications. Now some 30 years later, some current users of MUMPS systems include the U.S. Veterans Affairs system and the Harvard Community Health Plan.

The BICS is designed as an extended network with more than 60 "servers" (devices that collect, store, and publish information) and more than 3,000 user (client) workstations that provide information access and order entry. This latter function, physician order communication, was first launched in May 1993 and has achieved 100 percent house officer use for all orders. All this has been achieved in one of the busiest and most competitive academic institutions in Boston. But we are getting ahead of the story.

Staff Organization

The BICS has been in development for five years. The BWH information systems staff is divided among five working divisions:

- Systems development
- Technology planning
- Operations
- Management systems
- Center for Applied Medical Informatics

Systems Development

The systems development division consists of 30 staff dedicated to application programming. These system staffers have had a massive task, literally automating all but one ancillary department (radiology) along with providing all necessary nursing, physician, and management systems needs.

Technology Planning

The technology planning division consists of eight staff members who are involved with the ongoing "care and feeding" of the unique BICS information environment. Unlike the hardware and software maintenance workers in the BWH operations division, this group must stay at the leading edge of BWH information needs and determine the best way BICS can meet those needs.

Operations

The operations division consists of 30 staff members, two-thirds of whom are engaged in telecommunications services at BWH. The remainder are the dedicated runners throughout BWH who solve software and hardware problems with the system. Operations must add a new server approximately every three months to keep up with the information demands. (These server devices are IBM PS2-95s, with four gigabytes of disk storage per server.)

Management Systems

The management systems division of the BWH information systems department remains one of the keys to the success of BICS. The management systems group consists of 12 staff members who review admissions and long-range detailed studies to obtain the benefits of the daily data stream from BICS. This group provides the customized reporting and analysis that BWH leaders need on a regular basis to deal with the rapidly changing health care market in Boston, which by some estimates now is averaging 60 percent managed care.[11] With its management information group "closing the loop" for a data-based decision-making process, BWH is far ahead of many of its competitors that deal with retrospective information from nonintegrated systems.

Center for Applied Medical Informatics

The Center for Applied Medical Informatics at BWH, headed by Dr. Teich, was responsible for developing and implementing the physician order-entry portion of BICS, which was "turned on" in May 1994 and had handled more than 5 million physician orders through January 1, 1995. Dr. Teich and his team are responsible for the ongoing medical informatics research around the system, demonstrating the importance of the physician–computer connection in quantitative, "benchmarkable" ways that demonstrate the value of this system to every clinician, administrator, and managed care provider.

During our interview, Dr. Teich mentioned a particular pharmaceutical agent, high in cost and redundant in medical value with other less costly agents, that the BWH pharmacy had had problems encouraging physicians to stop prescribing. Using the order-entry portion of BICS, Dr. Teich and his team constructed an ordering pathway for physicians that, rather than controlling their behavior, spelled out alternative agents to this expensive drug and allowed the individual clinician to make a choice. The reported result was an 80 percent decrease in drug ordering over the time that the BICS pathways were put in place.[12] Such is an effective demonstration of closing the three-dimensional clinical information loop described in chapter 8. In fact, the rules-based reminder system built into BICS allows the laboratory, for example, to flag an abnormal value and actually have the system page the responsible physician to "8888." Everyone at BWH knows that means, "Sign on to one of the BICS terminals, doctor; I've got something important to tell you!"

Implementation and Maintenance

At the outset of the project, BICS was an inpatient ordering system only; however, an outpatient order-entry and results-reporting system was implemented in first quarter 1995. Several reasons account for the success of BICS.

First, house officer training takes only 45 minutes. The majority of house officer training occurs on the wards of BWH and employs nurses and other house officers as trainers. This kind of just-in-time training has been found to be most appealing to the house officers for the following reasons:

- It emphasizes the immediate benefits of using the system.
- It demonstrates the operational aspects of using the system as well as technical proficiency of system use.
- Having clinicians teach clinicians requires a lot less translation of user problems and issues, resulting in a much more efficient and effective training effort.

Second, BWH requires that a named clinician within the medical center own every rule on the BICS rules-based system. This is to ensure that as questions naturally arise as a result of BICS rules affecting clinical decision making, there is a recognized local expert who can explain the logic of the specific rule or guideline.

Third, there is close coupling between health services research, patient management services, and CIS at BWH. Health services research develops study protocols; patient management services works closely on fitting this to Joint Commission and other regulatory requirements; and BICS provides both the implementation methodology as well as the database recording the impact on physician-ordering behavior and patient outcomes.

It is quite clear that in Boston, the BWH system has been able to identify a common purpose of providing an integrated patient care information environment as a strategic tool for facing the rapid changes in U.S. health care. The physician–computer connection has clearly been a key component of that strategy.

Summary

This chapter has provided the reader with exemplars of the application of clinical decision support systems in U.S. health care today. The combination of enabling improvement in the quality of medical decision making *in balance* with decreasing the cost of care will be the final test of the value of clinical decision support systems as the end of this century approaches. Health care providers could do well to follow the lead of the pioneers described in this chapter.

References

1. Sittig, D., and Stead, W. W. Computer-based physician order entry: the state of the art. *Journal of the American Medical Informatics Association* 1(2):108–23, Mar.–Apr. 1994.

2. Johnston, M. E., Langton, K. B., Haynes, R. B., and Mathieu, A. Effects of computer-based clinical decision support systems on clinician performance and patient outcome: a critical appraisal of research. *Annals of Internal Medicine* 120(2):135–42, Jan. 15, 1994.

3. Johnston and others.

4. Wyatt, J., and Spiegelhalter, D. Field trials of medical decision-aids: potential problems and solutions. *Proceedings of the Annual Symposium in Computer Applications in Medical Care,* 1991, pp. 3–7.

5. Johnston and others.

6. Ogura, H., Sagara, E., Iwata, M., and others. Online support functions of prescription order system and prescription audit in an integrated hospital information system. *Medical Informatics* 13(3):161–69, July–Sept. 1988.

7. Berner, E. S., Webster, G. D., Shugerman, A. A., and others. Performance of four computer-based diagnostic systems. *New England Journal of Medicine* 330(25):1792–96, June 23, 1994.

8. Berner and others.

9. Weed, L. L. Knowledge coupling, medical education and patient care. *Critical Review Medical Informatics* 1(1):55–79, 1986.

10. Evans, R. S., and others. Improving empiric antibiotic selection using computer decision support. *Archives of Internal Medicine* 54:878–84, Apr. 25, 1994.

11. John Teich, MD, Director of Medical Informatics, Brigham and Women's Hospital, Boston. Personal communication with author, Jan. 10, 1996.

12. Teich.

Creating the Future: A Marriage of Technologies for Better Patient Care

The only thing that is constant is change. Few persons working in the health care field would take issue with that statement. Over the past 10 years, the three institutions discussed in this book—U.S. medicine, the U.S. health care system, and HCISs—have undergone tremendous change. This final chapter examines what changes are still likely to occur.

The trend in U.S. medicine appears to be a return by physicians to their earlier societal position. Subspecialization is no longer a mandate, and many young physicians are now encouraged to seek general practice positions. Furthermore, prepaid health plans, greater emphasis on health care cost containment, and the change in society's attitude toward authority figures all have transformed the average physician from an independent, authoritarian solo practitioner into today's staff physician.

The nature of medical practice is also slowly changing from an emphasis on the treatment of established disease toward preventive medicine. In this regard, physicians are taking important lessons from their European colleagues on the cost of preventing disease versus treating it only after diagnosis.

Outpatient care has changed to include modalities thought impossible or improper only a few years ago, including home labor and delivery, home IV therapy, and home mechanical ventilation. In fact, the emphasis of modern medicine is now on briefer in-hospital therapies and more care delivered in the outpatient setting. In concert with the enhanced mobility of society, many patients seek health care in many different settings—the physician's office, community clinics, emergency rooms, hospitals—making the coordination of care and information challenging.

Finally, although physicians still command a good deal of respect in our society, it is clear that the days of the unquestioned autocratic physician are over. Patients are demanding more information from their physicians and expect their physicians to work with them to arrive at effective treatment plans. These last two trends—the mobility of patients seeking care within different parts of the health care system, and the greater demand for the integration of that information—are special challenges for physicians in the coming decade.

U.S. hospitals are striving to adapt to significant financial and societal pressures to meet patient needs. For example, large inpatient facilities are disappearing in favor of women's pavilions featuring short-stay birthing rooms. Day-stay surgery has now become a way of life in all hospitals. Outpatient clinics are undergoing significant changes, erasing the busy, impersonal "inner-city" image of the past and becoming more like modern office settings. And, in a move for survival, hospitals are consolidating and forming hospital systems. This consolidation involves management, equipment, and all resources, including information. In fact, information resources (computers, technical staff, and so forth) sometimes are the catalysts in hospitals' consideration to move to higher levels of integration.

The days of U.S. hospitals acting independently of one another, duplicating costly procedures and equipment (for example, magnetic resonance imagers and positron-emission tomography scanners), are drawing to a close as a result of the changing medical financial scene. They will be replaced by centers similar to the Canadian specialty-based medical centers, where especially expensive or unique services are available to a network of other area hospitals through ambulance, helicopter, or even telecommunications linkage. These "hospitals without walls" will be available to smaller community hospitals, clinics, and offices. The successful health care system in the coming decades will involve networks of care delivery vehicles addressing society's health care needs with emphasis on cost-effective preventive care.

Consider the following scenario in this networked health care delivery system of the future: A patient is visiting his family physician at her office because of chest pains he suffered while working outside. The physician takes a history, performs a physical examination, and decides the patient should have both an electrocardiogram (ECG) and a chest X ray. Following those tests, the physician has some concerns about the patient's chest X ray and the ECG. Fortunately, she is connected to the regional health care system through her office information system terminal. Because both her office X-ray machine and ECG machine are equipped with computer outputs, both studies are instantly transmitted to an expert radiologist and cardiologist at the medical center 200 miles away. Through the video/telephone link, the physician discusses the case thoroughly and immediately with the consulting radiologist and cardiologist. Fortunately, the consensus is that the patient has not had a heart attack. However, the radiologist has detected signs of early smoking-related lung disease on the chest X ray. Counseling with his physician for smoking cessation and a bit of rest are all the patient will need for the moment.

Similarly, PCISs will continue to evolve into true patient-centered information networks that bear no resemblance to current systems. Although there are as many possible future directions for PCISs as there are futurists writing about them, the following major needs will be met one way or the other:

- Patient-centered health care databases
- Ergonomically correct, customized workstations
- Large-scale integration of health care system databases
- Full relational database structures
- Application of telecommunications technology to the practice of medicine
- Convenience of wireless computing
- Growth of interest in the World Wide Web
- Rise of the "patient–computer connection"

Patient-Centered Health Care Databases

As was discussed in an earlier chapter, the roots of HCISs have been in clerical and financial systems created and operated to support hospital operations. The organization of these systems is most often centered on a billable unit of care rather than a patient's medical history or clinical problems. As such, these databases become ineffective as patient care continuity tools. However, the changing environment of health care is driving us back to the roots of patient care and service, demanding a rethinking of institutional priorities and programs. The result is that what is best for patient care is now also best for the hospital's survival.

To best serve the patient, a PCIS must include the entire scope of clinical, financial, and operational data that define a patient's use of a health care system. A patient-centered database will include these elements and maintain continuity of the individual patient's information. Because the complexity of treating patients demands simultaneous access to all dimensions of a patient's care (medical, financial, demographic, and so forth), the information tool will have to present these data in an integrated and usable manner. Although special ways of combining the data and representing information have to be supported (see the following section), the most fundamental aspect of the information system's architecture and operation in the future will be its focus on the whole patient and his or her needs.

Customized Workstations

The more complex the PCIS, the more comprehensive the data that are electronically maintained, and the more human beings will need a "smart filter" to turn data into information. This is the purpose of the workstation. In the future, workstations will be powerful computers connected to larger information networks with full graphic, sound, and video as well as text presentation capabilities. Human interaction with these devices will vary from natural conversation to handwriting on an electronic pad to typewriter keyboards to pointing devices (including the one at the end of your arm). In addition to fulfilling its role as a PCIS terminal, the workstation will act as the X-ray review box, the ECG monitoring station, the electronic mail room, the video telephone, and the paging system.

In keeping with the special communication needs of different hospital users, the workstation needs to vary in size and shape. The nurse may soon have a workstation the size of a medical clipboard to take from room to room. Attached to it will be an automatic transducer for patient vital signs as well as a code reader for unit dosage of medications. House staff physicians may have prescription-pad-sized devices that also function as smart paging systems providing not only alerts but also the actual information on miniature high-resolution screens. Health care administrators may have workstations integrated into the tops of their desks that are as flat as ink blotters and about as large, continuously presenting hospital resource utilization information and communication facilities.

The most important aspect of workstations will be their functionality. Workstations in the future will present packets of patient information organized according to user-specified parameters. For example, the clinician will see information organized according to patient, diagnosis (to evaluate the correct diagnostic/therapeutic approaches), and provider. Information by provider will allow the clinician to evaluate his or her own performance in disease diagnosis and prescriptions according to a variety of outcome measurements: clinical, financial, and social. For example, clinicians will be able, on-line and in real time, to evaluate their own surgical morbidity and mortality by procedure, compare their costs per patient with those of other surgeons on staff and, finally, view the speed with which their patients return to work after surgery compared with other surgeons' patients. In this manner, the workstation acts as the most powerful QA tool possible.

For the health care executive, the workstation will allow real-time evaluation of hospital operations, including resource management, materials management, and financial performance. Decision support capabilities will allow the superimposition of models of management on current operations and permit on-the-fly strategic and tactical planning, including "what-if" scenarios, to improve the hospital's mission of providing patient care services. Ultimately, the workstation becomes the work environment as opposed to its current status as a supplement to that milieu.

Large-Scale Integration of Databases

So far, this chapter has discussed the integration of patient care information on the organizational and individual-user levels. However, the future of health care is directly tied to its ability to serve the needs of patients in an increasingly mobile society. Probably more than any other people, Americans exercise their freedom to travel and make choices. As stated previously, patients now seek health care in many diverse settings, including clinics, offices, and hospitals. The glue that will hold together these diverse sources of health care will be the large-scale integration of patient care databases.

For example, under such large-scale integration, the information network that serves a patient's care in hospital W would also be accessible through special security codes in hospital X, in clinic Y, and in physician's office complex Z. The current proliferation of paper records would be supplanted by the patient's electronic medical record, and it would be in the interests of all involved (patients, health care providers, institutions) to maintain this electronic record to provide the best continuity of care.

In such scenarios, one of the most common questions will be: Who owns and maintains this database? If you have been following the spirit of these future visions, you already know the answer to this question—the patient! With a credit-card-sized laser storage device known as a data card, patients will in fact be able to maintain possession and control of their health care records, simultaneously addressing concerns of security and mobility.

The large-scale integration of databases also involves information structures that support the hospitals-without-walls concept of networked HCISs throughout the country and the world. These linkages will progressively dissolve the need for reduplication of equipment and expertise in specialized, costly procedures and operations by making such resources available to any hospital and patient via satellite-linked networks. In the aforementioned example describing a patient experiencing chest pain, the diagnosis would likely be made with the help of a satellite-linked network to speed the transmission of both voice and picture data between the local physician's office and the medical center hundreds of miles away.

Full Relational Database Structures

The PCIS of the future will contain important information for the individual patient's care and follow-up. Additionally, with the electronic form of this information, cross-correlation of information between patients provides an ideal resource for clinical research and investigation as a by-product of patient care. Instead of the current expensive and labor-intensive process of advancing medical information through the multicenter trial, the judicious use of information within a PCIS can provide rapid insights into the effectiveness of various approaches to patient care and evaluation.

Among the most vexing limitations of the current medical research process are the following:

1. Clinical studies take a long time to complete.
2. The relevance of study results from one population of patients to another is not as great as might be expected.

3. The cost in time and money limits such research to only a small fraction of the number of clinical questions that need to be answered to really advance medical knowledge and the quality of patient care.

Although carefully constructed security measures must be in place, the data bank of clinical information contained in PCISs can be effectively used to address these limitations and provide cost-effective, rapid, and relevant clinical research to clinicians.

Full relational database structures give researchers access to such patient information as diagnosis, medication, and treatment across a number of institutions. For example, a full relational database would allow the following information to be retrieved using the *same* database:

1. The results of a patient's last five ECGs (data by patient)
2. The number of patients seen in a particular medical system in the past 10 years with the diagnosis of anterior myocardial infarction (data by diagnosis)
3. The number of patients seen in a particular medical system who are taking aspirin (data by medication)
4. The number of patients in a particular medical system who have undergone thrombolytic therapy in the past five years (data by treatment)
5. The number of patients seen in a particular medical center with the diagnosis of myocardial infarction, who are receiving aspirin and who have undergone thrombolytic therapy; and a list of the outcomes of intracranial or systemic bleeding (real-time clinical research)

Hospital administrators, medical insurance companies, and others would benefit from such information in making more informed decisions about medical liability, the cost of various treatments, and outcome management that makes sense, taking us out of our current practice of making our best guess on such important matters.

Telemedicine

In the past two years there has been a great deal of discussion about the connection between the "information highway" and medicine. In particular, telemedicine (the concept of using telecommunications technology in the delivery of health care) has become popular. In reality, telemedicine has been in existence since 1959, and there are already programs in more than 20 states and a number of foreign countries. Although a thorough discussion of telemedicine is outside the scope of this book, a few comments regarding the state of the art of telemedicine are relevant to the physician–computer connection.

Status Report

Although telemedicine has been around for 35 years, with well-developed programs in place (especially in Canada and Norway), telemedicine in the United States is still in its adolescence. In fact, some of the fundamental infrastructure, both technical and operational, has yet to be put in place in this country. Teleradiology, or the transmission of radiographs for remote interpretation and radiologic consultation, is still the most common form of telemedicine in the United States. Importantly, many academic medical centers are actively investigating the value of telemedicine to allow more cost-effective outreach of their consultative services. Programs investigating telesurgery, telepsychiatry, and other forms of teleconsultation are now under way. However, as discussed below, the standards for both equipment and support for this method of making the physician–computer connection are just entering into national debate, making most telemedicine efforts research by definition.[1]

Benefits

The literature is essentially devoid of prospective outcomes studies or health effectiveness research regarding telemedicine. This leaves most of the existing information descriptive or evaluative at best. However, a 1994 report on health care cost reductions estimated billions of dollars of savings by the effective institution of telemedicine communications via interconnection of the local access and transport areas between regional Bell telephone companies.[2] The following activities were proposed to effect those cost reductions:

* Reduction in patient transportation from rural to urban tertiary care centers by teleconsultation
* Delivery of medical information throughout a state's health care facilities, avoiding "orphan" remote sites
* Promulgation of standards of care and guidelines state and nationwide, decreasing malpractice costs
* Transfer of patient information intrastate and interstate without delay, allowing just-in-time CDS for our mobile population
* Delivery of health care information directly into patients' homes, providing the most cost-effective preventive health care information to the population directly

Research in Texas, Iowa, and other sites around the country will help determine the reality of these proposed benefits in the last half of this decade.

Impediments to the Growth of Telemedicine

There are a number of impediments to the growth of telemedicine in this country that will need to be carefully examined and dealt with if these new technologies are to fulfill their promise. These impediments include licensure, credentialing, confidentiality, and technology standards.[3]

Licensure for telemedicine suggests that a physician using the technology must be licensed in every state where the telecommunication link allows him or her to provide care. Considering the onerous current process of obtaining state licenses, this indeed may provide a limitation on the medium.

Credentialing for telemedicine is also part of the current tradition of granting physician "privileges" at a medical center prior to beginning practice. Telemedicine consultation, of course, could confound this tradition and therefore would need to be addressed prior to instituting telemedicine state- or nationwide.

Confidentiality has always posed a difficult problem in the physician–computer connection. The added dimension of telemedicine raises new questions, for the same technology that could move vital patient information across a state or across the nation could also be used, unknown to the patient, for unauthorized purposes. Hence, as we proceed to open up the medical information environment, we will be challenging our technology as never before to provide safeguards for information.

Technology standards provide yet another impediment to the growth of telemedicine. Currently there are many vendors of teleradiology systems. Unfortunately, most have developed completely proprietary solutions that do not allow easy sharing of radiographic material system to system. Likewise telecommunications and computerized patient information standards are needed to develop the regional and national medical record promised by the information highway. Therefore, although it is full of promise and at the vanguard of proposed benefits of the national information highway, telemedicine needs careful study before it can begin to fulfill its anticipated goal of providing a "virtual" health care information environment.

The State of the Art

The current state of the art of telemedicine can be summed up in the following consensus statements from a 1994 conference on telemedicine:[4]

- Focus on the needs of underserved people more than on the capabilities of available technologies and regional centers.
- Use the least expensive but appropriate telecommunications technology for any specific application.
- Telemedicine applications must be customized for each community and include as many uses of technologies as possible.

- Adequate training is essential during implementation of telemedicine (particularly if practitioners are to use it).
- Communications technology and availability can be very poor and a limiting factor in rural, and even urban, underserved areas.
- A decrease in a sense of isolation is a readily observable benefit of telemedicine extended to rural communities.
- The use of telecommunications to provide preventive health education to underserved populations may be as important as the actual improvement of care provided by means of telemedicine.
- When cost-effectiveness of new telemedicine systems and strategies is determined, value to the individual and the community is a critical consideration, and cost is only one element of the equation.
- Professional groups within the medical community should develop minimal technologic standards for telemedicine.
- All forms of telecommunication, not just high-end video systems, should be used in new telemedicine applications.
- Effective telemedicine will dramatically improve the ability of midlevel providers (for example, physicians' assistants and nurse practitioners) to participate in health care delivery to underserved populations.
- Telemedicine offers direct access to both traditional continuing medical education (CME) and "instantaneous" CME with every interaction between local and distant health care providers.
- As computer networks and other communications technologies develop, both their vertical and horizontal integration will be critical.
- Additional research on the quality of care achieved with telemedicine is needed.
- With the advent of advanced telecommunications technologies and the single national examination for medical licensure, current state-specific licensing should be reexamined.
- Jurisdictional issues related to malpractice and liability must be examined if telemedicine is to achieve a maximal effect on improved access to health care.
- Confidentiality with respect to medical records should be no more a problem with telemedicine than with other consultative practices.

Wireless "Personside" Computing

Wireless computing is undeniably one of the significant technologies of the 1990s, but what meaning does it hold for the physician–computer connection? Consider the following scenarios:

- Scenario #1: A busy attending surgeon has to perform rounds on the 12 patients for whom she is caring at a large community hospital. Her patients are scattered over four floors and it is 45 minutes before operating time begins. She needs the latest information on her patients and the ability to write orders immediately as she goes from bedside to bedside; otherwise, those orders will have to wait until this afternoon when the surgical cases are finished.

- Scenario #2: An internist begins his day planning to see 20 patients in a morning. He must move quickly from room to room in the four-room clinic area and must have at hand his previous dictated summaries as well as any outstanding labs and tests. There is little or no time to sit at a computer console and enter orders. He usually does his work literally between rooms, writing prescriptions and jotting down notes in the patient's presence. He and his partners have considered putting a computer in each exam room, but the expense is too high.
- Scenario #3: It is time to dispense medications at a busy pediatric ward. The charge nurse moves her med cart to the first room, and begins giving each patient his or her meds while checking on their conditions along the way. She marks her MEDS GIVEN sheet, which she will have to transcribe into the PCIS after she has finished dispensing meds. Nonurgent patient requests for change in diet, new pain medication, and so forth will have to wait until then as well.

In all these situations, the connection between clinician and computer is disrupted as a result of the demands of time and space in modern patient care. The standard implementation of a PCIS with stationary workstations simply does not take into account the required mobility of the modern physician and nurse who need patient information literally as they walk between patient rooms. The importance of this problem is evident when one considers that even the most intuitive, helpful PCIS will have little or no impact on the ordering physician if it is not used at the point of care.

Bedside computing is certainly not a new concept, but has failed to become a nationwide standard for PCIS implementations. There are a number of reported reasons for this: expense; reluctance of health care workers to spend more time at the patient's bedside documenting; and failure of the bedside paradigm to take into account the diversity of physical locations where health care workers gather, record, and use information.

Consider the following example illustrating the third reason. The ambulatory care physician quickly reviews his last notes on a patient he is about to see in his office. He then needs to contact the lab or radiology for the reports on recent tests. While in the patient's room, he reviews the therapeutic plan with the patient; after leaving the exam room, he writes out prescriptions and instructions for the patient and his records. It would seem that the failure of the desktop workstation to follow the clinician through his or her workday would be a serious barrier to delivering on the physician–computer connection. On the other hand, portable devices that deliver the power of the PCIS not to the bedside but to the person needing the information ("personside") could improve the connection significantly.

Fortunately, a number of evolving technologies are being applied to close this gap. These technologies may be categorized as the following:

- Dockable portable systems
- Limited-range wireless networks
- Long-range wireless communications

Long-range wireless communications technologies, including cellular communications, remain uncommon in health care applications. Although the portable cellular telephone market in the United States has exploded, and cellular, fax, and data transmission modems are now widely available, the use of cellular technology remains rare for PCIS implementation (although not for hospital paging telecommunications). Hence we will confine our comments to the dockable and limited-range wireless technologies.

Dockable Portable Systems

Dockable portable systems allow the clinician to have access to a suite of applications running directly on a portable device with complete freedom of mobility. The connection (or docking) with the main PCIS network occurs intermittently throughout the workflow either to pick up information from the network (for example, lab results, reports, and so on) or to send information into the network (such as orders, requests, and so forth). Such systems have been in production for several years.[5]

Advantages of such systems are as follows:

- They are completely portable.
- No radiofrequency (RF) or infrared (IR) transmissions are needed.
- Docking can occur when a break in workflow permits.
- Because there is no broadcast of information, security can be well maintained.

The limitations of such systems include the following:

- The connection with the PCIS network is intermittent and information may be needed ad hoc.
- Much of the PCIS application (at least the user interface) must reside wholly on the portable device, increasing the computational requirements for the device's power and display (thus increasing cost).
- The docking time in first- and second-generation systems remains slow, causing a bottleneck for information flow.

Limited-Range Technologies

Limited-range wireless networks are currently in use in health care applications throughout the United States. The University of West Virginia is one such example, where a wireless network throughout the medical center handles all communications to and from the centralized integrated PCIS. Over the past year, improving technologies in IR networks have improved the performance and decreased the need for direct "line-of-sight" connection between the roving portable device and the IR base unit (diffuse IR).

The advantages of such systems are as follows:

- Real-time connection with the PCIS network, allowing interactive information query and data transmission
- In the case of IR technology, inexpensive wireless technology that will be built into the next generation of personal computers
- Good fit with most health care applications where information is collected and transmitted within a defined area (such as ambulatory clinic, office, inpatient ward, and so on)

Disadvantages are unfortunately considerable:

- Recent growing concern over the health risks of radiofrequency irradiation[6] raises questions of applicability of at least RF technology in health care.
- Infrared technology, although less dependent on line of sight, still cannot penetrate walls and doors, making some implementations, such as clinic offices, very problematic.
- Cost of RF technology is still quite high and competition for remaining RF spectra has now become a financial boon for the current administration in Washington.
- Power requirements for the wireless network technology (especially RF) remain high, adding battery life concerns.
- Because information is broadcast by both RF and IR technologies, the risk of information interception and security violations has been raised.
- In general, the most useful technology, RF, is still in its infancy and the most embattled by both political (spectra limitations) and health issues.

Although these technologies for wireless personside computing hold tremendous promise, they remain in a current state of flux without standards and a clear dominant methodology today. This, however, has not abated the demand for such systems and there are a growing number of institutions throughout the United States applying IR and RF technologies in daily practice (for example, Maine Medical Center, Portland, Maine; Trippler Medical Center, Honolulu; and others).

Bottlenecks in Technology Deployment

An issue common to all forms of portable, wireless technology is the type of personal device that will deliver the information to the clinician. Although electronics have been considerably miniaturized over the past 10 years, the demands of a PCIS test the very best of the available technologies. Specifically, display technology and power supply technology remain bottlenecks to the rapid growth of wireless PCIS computing. The advantages of graphic user interfaces (GUIs) are now an established fact. They appear to be especially useful when navigating large amounts of information as required in health care. As an example, note the significant increase in the use of the Internet since the introduction of graphically oriented software such as Mosaic. Unfortunately, portable display technology has only recently provided adequate color and resolution to make these GUIs usable. Furthermore, the current power requirements of the best portable display technologies significantly affect battery life. It is safe to say that the power and display requirements of emerging client/server technologies will continue to push the limits.

Fortunately, research throughout the world that will address these issues is intense, with breakthroughs expected in the very near future. Already, fully configured portable laptop computers that until one year ago could not be expected to keep working for more than one or two hours can reliably go eight hours between charges. With the increasing changes in health care delivery and the mobility of our society, it is fairly certain that the application of innovative technologies in the portable wireless network arena will come fast and furious over the last half of this decade.

The World Wide Web

The entire field of informatics has been vastly changed in the past two years with the building of the information highway, known as the Internet. Although this book is not a technology manual, the Internet is far too important a change in the international informatics landscape for us to ignore it. The Internet has allowed a common information network link to be possible within a medical center, within a town, in a region, or between sites around the world—all in real time. Previously such a level of communication using private networks was either extremely expensive or not available at all.

Furthermore, the advent of the World Wide Web has resulted in the creation of a de facto standard of information collection and presentation using browsers. These software programs have already been developed for essentially every type of personal computer platform in use. Obviously this degree of common information access and sharing is entirely unprecedented with one exception: the telephone. Perhaps the most relevant comparison is between the telegraph and the telephone.

Prior to the common availability of the telephone, telegraph operation was a skill restricted to a few (sometimes only one individual in an entire town) acting as the information link. Once it became possible for people to simply speak into a mouthpiece and be heard from coast to coast, the telegraph's fate was sealed. Similarly, although enjoying significant growth, the personal computer revolution has been perceived as the creation of "islands" of information, much like the history of hospital-based CISs. From an information technology perspective, the Internet and the Web have already converted the world from information islands into a single, large, interlinked continent. Only time will tell how this finally transmutes the face of health care technology.

The purpose of this section is to: (1) provide some basic understanding of the Internet, (2) identify the significance of the Internet for the clinical information expert and physician, (3) highlight the key elements of the Internet that will have the most relevance for CISs, and (4) introduce some of the most important concerns about this new world of global information communication.

Some Definitions

Outside the medical profession, few areas have generated new jargon faster than the Internet. For the reader to begin to understand the importance of the Internet, some definitions are essential.

An *internet* (lower case "i") is little more than a network linking networks together. The *Internet* (upper case "I") is nothing less than the grandmother of all networks, linking networks together literally around the globe. These linked networks include commercial, university, military, and other research networks. The Internet is growing at a phenomenal rate, with more than 20 million Americans using it daily at the time of this writing.[7] The Internet involves moving information using "the Internet protocol," which makes it possible for so many people, computers, and networks all to be working as if they were one.

The *World Wide Web* (WWW, or simply Web) is a method of navigating all the networks on the Internet. The Web uses a method of connecting information on the Internet called *hypertext*, wherein one can jump from one bit of information to another by means of links. The Web runs via a software program called a *browser* (brand names include Netscape and Mosaic) that graphically displays these links as highlighted text. To jump to the connected information, one simply clicks on the highlighted text with a pointing device such as a mouse. The growth in use of the Internet has been directly related to the availability of the Web, making Internet navigation easy and even fun. In fact, using the Web to find information on the

Internet is called "surfing"! The Web is programmed in hypertext markup language (HTML). More recently, progress has been made in allowing navigation on the Internet using a three-dimensional graphic representation of cyberspace called *virtual reality markup language* (VRML).

Most recently, the term *Intranet* has appeared, describing the use of Internet and Web technology in smaller "private" networks. The Intranet provides some of the advantages of these technologies while supplying an enhanced degree of security for sensitive information. That aspect is particularly relevant in the health care field.

Advantages for Physicians

The key benefits of the Internet and Web for physicians are: (1) ease of use; (2) de facto standards for linking to patients, other physicians, providers, and so forth; (3) integration of information access; and (4) geographic access independence.

The Web browser has become one of the fastest growing segments of the international software market in a decade. The same skill that allows individuals to read a printed page allows them to read and use a Web browser. The interface is intuitive and uncluttered, and actually requires little personal computing power to execute, as most of the intelligence is located in the Internet network, not the personal computer. From the time the Web was first developed, on-line help links were used extensively to minimize the need for training and manuals. Nevertheless, the increasing complexity of clinical information retrieval and analysis taxes even the best of the current Web offerings. However, with the advent of new Web programming environments such as Java, these limitations should soon be overcome.

With more than 20 million Americans using the Web daily, there's a good chance that physicians will be able to find not only their colleagues on-line but their patients as well! Recent research has suggested that patients with chronic illnesses may actually prefer the Web as a means of accessing frequently asked questions and nonurgent advice from health care professionals to traditional means such as the telephone or office visit. Several articles have already appeared in the medical literature demonstrating the possibilities of direct physician–patient communication links using Internet technology.[8-13]

With its rapid growth, the Web has provided an unprecedented means of information integration. The pressure for vendors to facilitate information access via Web tools is significant, thereby creating de facto standards of information interchange and potentially lowering the costs of system development. Fortuitously, previously slowly evolving CISs such as HL7 have been reenergized by the growth of the Web, enabling the clinician to access data from multiple systems via "interface engines."[14]

Finally, access to the Web has now taken on an entirely new dimension with the entry of large telecommunications carriers such as AT&T and MCI into the Internet connection market. Whereas the early history of the Internet had involved a multiplicity of smaller networking companies, now the same giants that built the telephone empire are rushing toward Internet cyberspace ("cyber" means "steering or control"). As of this writing, there remains an ongoing competition between cable television and telecommunications industry leaders as to who will be the "standard" provider of Internet access. In any event, the individual user is the winner, as costs for connectivity are plummeting weekly and the pressure to maintain speed of access and ease of use remains strong and steady. In fact, it may soon cost less than $200 per access point to the Internet, with monthly charges of $18 or less—similar to the average telephone bill.

Access to the Web

Regarding access to the Web, a common criticism from physicians is, "It seems to be so disorganized, I can't really find anything I need!" The problem here largely stems from the way in which the Internet is organized. Information is distributed throughout the Internet, and, until fairly recently, there were few sources that pulled together specific information. That has changed, however; literally every day more information resource collections specifically targeted toward the health care field are becoming available on the "Net." Different information areas on the Internet have universal resource locators (URLs), or "addresses;" by simply typing in the correct address, the user can go directly to the desired information area. Following is a collection of Internet sites specifically directed toward medicine, including their URLs:

- http://www.med.umich.edu/ The University of Michigan (one of the pioneers of the Internet) Medical Centers Frontpage:, regularly updated pointers to other topics of medical interest throughout the Internet. Physician- and patient-oriented information are contained within pediatric psychiatry, transplantation, and pediatric cardiology sections.
- http://www.nih.gov/ National Institutes of Health NIH Homepage; connection to news and events, grants information, health information resources including AIDS information, and a listing of published clinical practice guidelines.
- http://www.nlm.nih.gov/ National Library of Medicine Homepage, HyperDOC provides a method of navigating the Web by linking to many varied medical information resources, including medical graphics and animations.
- http://biomed.nus.sg/Cancer/welcome.html Homepage of the National Cancer Institute; providing information from the physicians data query

(PDQ) reference on the latest chemotherapy protocols in the treatment of cancer.

- http://cancer.med.upenn.edu/ OncoLink at the University of Pennsylvania with additional information on recent research and clinical information in oncology.
- http://indy.radiology.uiowa.edu/VirtualHospital.html Homepage of The University of Iowa College of Medicine's Virtual Hospital, one of the first (and still one of the best) multimedia demonstrations of clinical information on the Web.

Although it will be several more years before the full ramifications of connection between the Internet and the physician will become clear, it is apparent that synergy will occur. For example, although there are few commercial resources that could deliver on a true nationwide electronic medical information resource, the Internet is already in place, linking people daily around the globe. Concerns about information security are important but not insoluble; therefore, the Internet may be the first version of an actual national information highway.

Finally, an interesting evolution of Internet browser software is now occurring. Because the Internet is a de facto standard, commercial software companies are now building new program development tools around Internet access. Because the Internet already handles multimedia information (albeit limited), the Internet software explosion may pave the way for the multimedia electronic medical record that seemed only "vaporware" just a few years ago. In short, the Internet is a new, invigorating aspect of the Information Age, and those responsible for making the physician–computer connection might well be advised to "get on the Net" and learn more about this phenomenon firsthand.

Confidentiality Concerns

Already the popular press has begun amplifying the paranoia of patient record leaks via unsecured transmission over the Internet with dire consequences for the patient/victim, including loss of job and insurance and worse. Patient information confidentiality and security, however, is indeed a real concern that needs to be understood and championed by physicians and other health care information professionals.

To say that technology may be used for good or ill is a cliché. However, the rapid entry of society onto the information highway now is beginning to reveal a dark side to information availability. Our responsibility as health care information professionals in the Information Age is to ensure that our patients' trust cannot be broken by electronic "hacking" or other espionage. Technology is already providing some answers with encryption, intranets, and "firewalls" (electronic barriers between sensitive information and the outside international networks). However, the real price of this emerging information access is vigilance. It would be just as irresponsible today for a physician to transport confidential patient information over an unencrypted E-mail communication as it would have been to leave a patient's written record open in the middle of the hospital cafeteria in the past. Many health care professionals are unaware of these issues, however, making all the more urgent the need for education and sensitization of staff to the threats as well as benefits that the newest technologies can bring to the delivery of health care.

Importance of Physician Involvement

From every perspective—cost of care, delivering on the health care system "without walls," remaining at the forefront of patient information accuracy, confidentiality, and security—we as health care information professionals must better understand this new era of information technology. Although many texts already crowd the bookshelves on the topic of the Internet, clearly the best way for physicians to understand the Web is to begin to use it themselves. Now with step-by-step packages from myriad sources, that process is easier than it has ever been. It is essential that physicians bring the same energy and dedication to understanding and advocating for the proper use of the information highway as we have been advocates for the quality of our patients' care in the past.

The Patient–Computer Connection

The 1990s could arguably be labeled the "health and fitness" decade in the United States. The interest in personal health has ballooned in this country in every aspect of daily life, from the spread of health food stores to sales of all varieties of home exercise equipment. Self-help in health care also has become more popular, with the void left by traditional health care being filled by practitioners of preventive medicine. It should come as no surprise, therefore, that a new dimension of health care computing, the patient–computer connection, is becoming increasingly important.

The patient–computer connection can perhaps be best described by the following vision:

- Every man, woman, and child in this country can easily access information relevant to preventing illness in themselves and their family.
- Everyone can access reparative health care information 24 hours a day, seven days a week, as needed, without the barriers of the current health care establishment.
- Patients can access, correct, update, and control access to their own electronic health care record.

Early efforts at developing this patient–computer connection were launched in the late 1980s, when electronic bulletin boards were used in Boston as a surrogate for physician office calls. Patients would simply sign on to a group practice's electronic bulletin board, review the on-line frequently asked questions (FAQs), and receive a response within 24 hours online from one of the physicians who staffed the bulletin board during his or her off-hours.

The practice of patient-generated histories is not a new idea. The notion is simply to allow patients to carefully and completely define their health care problem with passive or active prompting from a health care professional. However, few clinics capitalize on this strategy better than the Given Health Clinic at the University of Vermont in Burlington. Based on their presenting complaint, patients receive color-coded history questionnaires, the responses to which constitute the basis for the face-to-face interview process with the clinic physician. Subsequently this information is captured into a computer database. The patient-generated information is then coded and easily retrieved for quality, practice review, and many other purposes. Benefits to this approach are multiform:

- Patients' real concerns can be most accurately captured.
- Patients' beliefs about their vulnerability to health care problems can be revealed.
- Patients take an active, vigorous role in the health care process.
- The accuracy of the clinical information is often superior when patients are encouraged to document their own histories.

The Hearth program at the University of Michigan is another example of the patient–computer connection in practice. It is designed around the concept of the hearth as the traditional center of family discussion and comfort. Patients with oncologic diseases regularly sign on through the Internet to their nurse clinicians and physicians via E-mail. They then personally search the relevant databases, presenting alternative protocols to their treating physicians gleaned from databases from around the world. It is interesting that physicians receiving input from their patients on these topics have actually welcomed the input rather than been threatened or angered by their patients' participation in what had previously been considered medical decision making.

Certainly these early efforts at developing the patient–computer connection are not the full vision of telemedicine with remote communications, diagnoses, and treatments that have been promised in so many health care vendor vision demonstrations. Rather we are seeing the transition from a paternalistic/maternalistic health care environment to one in which there is far more empowered patient involvement. We are witness to an era in which the information necessary to prevent disease is moved directly to the place where it is needed most, the home and the individual.

Physician Use of New Technologies

The aforementioned new technologies should have a major impact on physician involvement in, and use of, PCISs. Because medical decision making is a complex process that integrates elements of many disciplines (clinical diagnosis, medical research, epidemiology, biostatistics, finance, and so forth), physicians require the highest sophistication in their information tools (for example, computers), first to assist and then to enhance their ability to carry out their professional activities.

The medical information explosion has made it impossible for clinicians to both keep track of all important medical developments and maintain a busy clinical practice. It is probable that this situation will continue for the foreseeable future and may even worsen. Therefore, physicians will always require the most advanced technology to cope with the increasing complexity of their profession. To be effective, the health care industry also must keep pace with this complexity. But how will physicians become involved in setting the requirements for these new technologies, and who will be responsible for informing them?

Two major groups will assume responsibility for involving more physicians in health care technology and informing them of new advances: health care information managers and physicians trained in applied medical informatics.

Health Care Information Management

Health care information managers are CIOs, vice presidents of information systems, data processing directors, and others who have recognized the key role that physicians can play in the successful selection, design, implementation, and use of PCISs for their institutions. These individuals have realized the strategic and tactical advantages of including physicians in this process. For example, strategic planning for consolidation of several small hospitals into a single medical center will occur with much greater speed and ease if there is a successful PCIS operating at the "mother" hospital that is in demand by the medical staffs of the satellite institutions.

Tactically, a medical center with physicians effectively using a PCIS has an excellent instrument for the introduction of QA or total quality management initiatives via the staffwide communications capabilities of the system. It is nearly impossible today to attend a health care professionals convention that does not have a distinct information systems track. Hence, health care professionals will continue to demand more involvement from physicians in PCISs to achieve maximum benefits from their health care dollar investment.

Medical informatics has been in existence for more than 30 years and has resulted in an impressive body of literature and research. That has given rise to many technological advances that have created the infrastructure for the modern-day PCIS. Major universities both in the United States and abroad have developed informatics departments that continue to provide an invaluable testing ground for the development of the latest information technologies. Yet several nationally recognized medical informatics experts have recently noted the slow growth of medical informatics departments in the United States and the failure of informatics to attract more clinically oriented physicians.

Physicians Trained in Applied Medical Informatics

In light of the existing academic infrastructure of medical informatics and the increasing need for clinical information tools in daily clinical practice, it would seem the ideal time to nurture a new subspecialty of medicine called applied medical informatics (AMI). This is a method of directly addressing the need to involve clinicians in medical informatics by making the subspecialty a recognized part of mainstream clinical medical training.

The relationship between the current medical informatics establishment and AMI is analogous to the two well-recognized divisions within medical disciplines of primary or "bench" researchers and clinical researchers. *Bench research* is the realm of physician–scientists and consists primarily of laboratory research. *Clinical research* is usually directed primarily toward investigations of clinical practice, including trials of new treatments and medications. Whether AMI exists as a subdivision of existing medical informatics departments or a division of clinical departments is not as important as the orientation and influence that graduates, themselves practicing clinicians, will have on their peers to more effectively inform physicians of new information tools and the best methods of application to day-to-day practice. Discussion of AMI is currently a common topic at national medical informatics conventions such as the Society for Computer Applications in Medical Care (SCAMC).

Summary

The future of health care is intimately connected with the future of PCISs. If the current pressures on the clinical and administrative systems in health care bring physicians and hospital managers closer together to improve patient care, the future will be bright indeed. In this book, we have attempted to provide the guideposts and architectures for forging better information tools to facilitate this collaboration. Only through close collaboration between clinicians and health care information professionals can a truly effective patient care information infrastructure be designed, developed, and implemented. We hope these tools will make it easier for you to achieve your goals.

References and Notes

1. Tangal, E. G. Testimony before Subcommittee on Investigations and Oversight on Science, Space and Technology. U.S. House of Representatives, May 21, 1994.

2. Healthcare Cost Reductions: The InterLATA Component. Boston: Arthur D. Little, 1994.

3. Sanders, J. H. Telemedicine: bringing medical care to isolated communities. *Journal of the Medical Association of Georgia* 82:237–41, May 1993.

4. McGee, R., and Tangalos, E. *Clinical Proceedings* 69:1131-36, May 1994.

5. Puritan Bennett, Pleasanton, CA.

6. Zhao, Z., Zhang, S., Zho, H., Zhang, S., Su, J., and Li, L. The effects of radiofrequency (<30 Mhz) radiation in humans. *Reviews on Environmental Health* 10(3-4):213-15, Jul.–Dec. 1994.

7. http://www.nlm.nih.gov/publications/staff__publications/rodgers/internet__ course/growth.html

8. Kassirer, J. P., and Angell, M. The Internet and the journal. *New England Journal of Medicine* 332(25):1709-10, June 22, 1995.

9. Chi-Lum, B. I., Lundberg, G. D., and Silberg, W. M. Physicians accessing the Internet, the PAI project: an educational initiative. *JAMA* 275(17):1361-2, May 1, 1996.

10. Yom, S. S. The Internet and the future of minority health. *JAMA* 275(9):735, Mar. 6, 1996.

11. Doyle, D. J. Surfing the Internet for patient information: the personal clinical web page. *JAMA* 274(20):1586, Nov. 22-29, 1995.

12. Glowniak, J. V., and Bushway, M. K. Computer networks as a medical resource: accessing and using the Internet. *JAMA* 271(24):1934-39, June 22-29, 1994.

13. Goldwein, J. W., and Benjamin, I. Internet-based medical information: time to take charge. *Annals of Internal Medicine* 123(2):152-53, July 15, 1995.

14. "Interface engines" are now common in the health care industry. For a detailed discussion see URL:http://www.ibm.com.au/IndSolu/health/iet.html

Anatomy of Information Technology Departments: A Primer for the Physician Champion

Modern health care information technology (IT) organizations are complex structures. Although it is not necessary for the physician champion to have an MBA degree, understanding the type of organization he or she is working with is important in determining the most likely path toward successful design, selection, and implementation of a PCIS. IT functional organizations can be categorized into vertical and horizontal models, with the latter subdivided into federations and confederations. For each of these models, this section reviews (1) basic description ("diagnosis"), (2) functional definition ("physiology"), and (3) successful strategies ("therapeutic plan and prognosis").

It is important to keep in mind that a particular organization may either be successful and functional or completely dysfunctional with any one of these models operative. Simply put, the kind of IT organizational model is no guarantee of operational success. Depending on your style as a physician champion (or CIO supporting such a champion), you may be more comfortable and individually successful with one kind of IT structure than another.

The Vertical Organization

Diagnosis

The vertically structured IT organization may be thought of as the authoritarian model or centralized model. This organization is recognizable by the manner in which decisions are made, namely top-down. If the question "Who makes the decisions around here?" repeatedly receives the same names in answer, the organization is probably vertically structured. This kind of IT organization is usually quite proud of displaying hierarchical organizational charts with boxes defining every person within the organization. They may even be posted throughout the department.

Physiology

The vertical-model IT organization may be successful or not, depending on key management leadership; however, it may be argued that enlighted management would not allow a purely vertical, centralized decision-making process to exist. An exception to this may be an IT organization in a small community hospital where a vertical decision model would exist by necessity. If the physician champion is aligned with the IT leader, then apparent communication efficiency and effectiveness may result.

Therapeutic Plan and Prognosis

In many ways, the vertical model of an IT organization is familiar to the practicing physician. The traditional physician role in medicine is top-down and authoritarian in many ways. Although the concept of the health care team is changing that role somewhat, in most health care settings (particularly office practices) the vertical support model still is alive and well. However, some would describe this kind of vertical structure as much more analogous to a NASA spaceship launch team rather than a military dictatorship. In the former all work toward the success of the astronauts as a team; in the latter, individual efforts lose importance to the glory of the dictator. It is hoped that the NASA model is the one most familiar to most physician champions.

Clearly the path to success in the vertically structured organization depends on the relationship between the physician champion and the IT leader (the CIO). Communication between these two individuals must flow easily and may greatly simplify decision making and expedite planning. However, the dependency on a few individuals also has serious shortcomings for the health care organization being served. For example, if a CIO leaves an organization (not an uncommon occurrence with an average CIO term of less than three years in the United States), then the physician champion will need to spend time completely redeveloping relationships, projects, and plans with a new administration. If a busy CIO is frequently unavailable, important decisions may be delayed, and if unexpected events arise, there is little resilience in the organization to respond to urgent needs.

There is an additional caveat for the physician champion regarding the vertical organization. All too often, the IT organization's true leadership is the financial department. As discussed in previous chapters, this is often a historical relationship between generating bills in a fee-for-service medical environment and the need for computers to help keep up with the many rules and regulations that must be met to be a financially successful health care organization. However, if the CFO is indeed the CIO, then the conflict between PCIS needs and financial information systems needs will perforce be greater than if the IT leadership is directly responsible to the CEO alone.

Experience indicates that this conflict does arise from both the high cost of CISs and the need for clinical system infrastructure, both of which compete with the needs of most institutions' busy financial services function. As noted in chapter 8, this conflict will likely change little in the new era of managed care.

Therefore, although the vertically organized IT structure may greatly simplify the communication work process, there is a significant price to pay for this apparent simplicity.

The Horizontal Organization

Diagnosis

The horizontally structured IT organization may also be described as the distributed model or decentralized model. The horizontal IT organization may be recognized by the existence of a number of "decision-making bodies" that may include individuals from within and outside the formal IT structure, charged with the responsibility of making IT decisions and setting priorities. In several recent excellent reviews, issues in health care IT governance have been raised illucidating the connection between current directions in structure of IT organizations and their function. One paradigm identifies IT organizations as functional federations or confederations.[1,2] This subcategorization of a horizontal IT model significantly clarifies the nature of this kind of structure.

Physiology

A federation is defined as the formation of a political unity, with a central government, by a number of separate states. From an IT perspective, a federation is a governance structure in which strategic decisions, such as those regarding major directions and services, are made by a central authority. The tactical decisions, however (for example, how to forward the strategic initiatives) are left to IT project groups with the responsibility and authority to get the job done. In this way, a federation IT model is a sort of hybrid: part vertical in its strategic decision making, part horizontal in its tactical project implementation.

A confederation is defined as an alliance or league. From an IT perspective, a confederation is a governance structure in which individual groups make both strategic and tactical decisions. This confederated horizontal system often results in significant duplication of efforts, increased cost of IT as a result of duplication and lack of a consistent direction, and, obviously, low productivity of the IT organization as a whole.

Therapeutic Plan and Prognosis

From the foregoing definitions, it would appear that a physician champion could effectively negotiate a federation horizontal organization, but would likely fail to be successful in a confederation. In a federation, provided the physician champion was included in the centralized strategic governance body, he or she could be effective in communicating clinicians' needs and the proper introduction of PCISs. In a confederation, however, the champion would have to lobby every decision-making body within IT and hope the majority would agree with the suggested direction and approach. Even if that type of success were possible, however, without central coordination, a confederation would still likely fail to implement a successful PCIS effort because of the inevitable disintegrating stresses that arise as a by-product of major enterprisewide projects. Therefore, it would be well for the new physician champion to evaluate the IT organization he or she is about to enter to ensure that its modern decentralized structure works far more as a federation of states than a confederated league.

Role of the Physician Champion in IT Governance

We have reviewed the anatomy and physiology of some models of IT organizations in the hopes of orienting the physician champion to the potential advantages and disadvantages that he or she may experience while in the role of physician leader. We also present this information to allow new physician champions the opportunity to evaluate the effectiveness of their institution's IT organization. Although most organizations exist as a hybrid, with authority centralized for some elements and distributed for others, it is often the nature and strength of the relationship between the CIO and the physician champion that determines the effectiveness of the ultimate outcome, the achievement of the physician–computer connection.

References

1. Strosberg, M. A. Technology and the governance of the health care industry: the dilemma of reform. *Journal of Health Politics, Policy and Law* 2(2):212–26, Summer 1977.

2. Levine, H. S., and Chaloner, R. S. Redefining the information technology governance model for an integrated delivery system. *Healthcare Information Management* 9(4):23–30, Fall 1995.

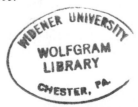